THE MMS HANDBOOK

Antje Oswald M.D.

The MMS Handbook

Your Health in Your Hands

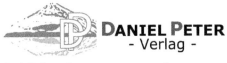

Publisher for a new consciousness

Copyright © 2015 Daniel Peter Verlag, Schnaittach, Germany

All rights reserved. This book or parts thereof may only be reproduced or copied with the prior written permission of the publisher. The same applies for the distribution of the book in mechanical, eletronic or audio form.

Translation from the German Dr Seiriol Dafydd

Editing / Proofreading Dr Rhiannon Ifans

Layout Monika Wolf

Typesetting Hans-Jürgen Maurer

Cover image Christiane Brendel, 'Vom Anfang' [Of the Beginning], 2005, acrylic on muslin, 100 x 120 cm

Publisher Daniel-Peter-Verlag, Schnaittach, Germany

Email info@daniel-peter-verlag.de

Phone number for orders 0049 (0) 9126 298 62 99

Internet www.daniel-peter-verlag.de

First English edition 2016
Translated from the fifth German edition 2014

ISBN 978-3-9815255-3-3

We welcome inquiries from international publishers regarding the publication of this book in translation.

Legal Disclaimer

The procedures explained in this book serve as information only. They do not replace medical diagnosis, advice or treatment.

Neither the author nor the publisher is responsible for damages of any kind resulting from the use of methods described in this book. We expressly do not accept responsibility for any improvement or deterioration in your state of health.

Due to the dynamics of the internet, links mentioned in the book that were active as the book went to press may now have changed, or may no longer be available.

Acknowledgements

I am grateful to Jim Humble for being so ready to share his knowledge of MMS with me and for answering all my questions. I would also like to thank Mia Hamel and Jenny Kimberley, Jim Humble's personal assistants, who supplied the required information.

Dr Paul John helped me to become familiar with the fundamentals of the chemistry of MMS, which made work much easier for me. My heartfelt thanks.

My sincere thanks too to my publisher who supported me in any and every way possible, and to Monika Wolf and Hans-Jürgen Maurer who designed the book so beautifully.

Dr Hartwin von Gerkan agreed to read the manuscript and made a number of valuable suggestions. Many thanks.

Over the last 20 years, Brigitte and Wolfgang Schiefer have given me numerous practical tips regarding wholefood diets, building biology, and geomancy, and have thereby contributed to making this the book it is.

Many thanks too to Alexander Praetorius for his constructive criticism.

Particular thanks are due to my colleague Kerstin Depping for her patience in typing my manuscripts, which were not easy to decipher.

I thank my mother, my father, my family and my teachers who made it possible for me to develop independently and to bravely walk new paths. I also thank my patients and those who have attended my courses for the trust they have placed in me.

I am indebted to all who sent in experience reports for this book, especially Ann Schneider-Cullen and Lothar Paulus who sent in numerous reports.

My deep-felt gratitude goes to my partner Christiane, who encouraged me with loving serenity, and in doing so provided vital support for body and mind through the highs and lows of writing this book. She also provided her beautiful image 'Vom Anfang' [Of the Beginning] for the book cover.

Many thanks to you all!

Contents

Foreword by Jim Humble 11
Foreword to the Expanded Edition 12
Introduction 13

1	**How it all began**	15
2	**The study and discovery of MMS**	19
3	**Mode of action**	23
4	**Remarkable therapeutic successes**	30
4.1	Experience reports from Belgium, Denmark, Germany, Great Britain, Austria, Switzerland and Mexico	34
4.1.1	Experience reports from self-responsible users	34
4.1.2	Experience reports from animal owners	81
5	**How to get hold of MMS**	92
6	**How to use MMS**	95
6.1	Preparing and taking MMS	96
6.2	Acid–alkaline balance	103
6.2.1	Adding sodium bicarbonate to neutralise, stabilise and improve the taste	104
6.3	The new standard protocol: MMS 1000 protocol	106
6.4	Jim Humble's former standard protocol	108
6.5	Clara's 6+6 protocol	108
6.6	MMS for pregnant women	109
6.7	MMS for infants	109
6.8	MMS for children	111
6.9	Slow activation based on the Fischer method	112
6.10	Who should take particular care when taking MMS?	113
6.11	Contraindications	114
6.12	Possible responses to MMS	115
7	**What to do if adverse reactions occur**	118
8	**More ways of administering MMS**	121
8.1	Sprayed onto the skin	121
8.2	Bathing with MMS	123

8.3	Brushing teeth and mouth washing with MMS	125
8.4	MMS enemas	126
8.5	MMS foot baths	128
8.6	MMS eye drops	129
8.7	MMS in intravenous infusions	130
8.8	Nasal inhalation of MMS	133
8.9	Cleansing spaces with MMS	135
8.10	Using MMS in a gas bag	135
8.11	Disinfecting water	137
8.12	Disinfecting food	138
8.13	Chlorine dioxide solution (CDS)	139
8.14	Gefeu solution	144
8.15	MMS energy globules	148
9	**MMS 2**	150
10	**DMSO and MMS**	154
11	**Safety instructions for the use of MMS, ClO$_2$, CDS, MMS 2 and DMSO**	160
11.1	Handling MMS safely	161
11.2	Handling hydrochloric acid safely	163
11.3	Handling tartaric acid safely	163
11.4	Handling citric acid safely	164
11.5	Handling chlorine dioxide solution safely	164
11.6	Handling MMS 2 safely	165
11.7	Handling DMSO safely	166
12	**Dosage recommendations for patients with various illnesses**	167
	AIDS	167
	Allergies	168
	Alzheimer's disease	168
	Apoplexy	168
	Arteriosclerosis	169
	Arthritis	169
	Asthma	171
	Atopic dermatitis	171
	Back pains	172
	Basal cell carcinoma	173
	Burns	173

	Cancer	174
	Children's diseases	177
	Colds	177
	Coxsackievirus	177
	Diabetes	177
	Excess weight	178
	Eye diseases	179
	Flu (including Swine flu)	179
	Heart diseases	181
	Hepatitis A, B, C, and other hepatitis types	181
	Herpes	182
	High blood pressure	182
	HIV *see* AIDS	182
	Hypertension *see* High blood pressure	182
	Injuries	182
	Lyme disease	183
	Malaria	184
	Melanoma	185
	MRSA	185
	Multiple sclerosis (MS)	187
	Parkinson's disease	187
	Severe illnesses	187
	Skin cancer	188
	Skin diseases of all kinds	188
	Sleep disorders	188
	Stomach ulcers	189
	Stroke *see* Apoplexy	189
	Sunburn	189
	Swine flu *see* Flu	189
	Tinnitus	189
13	**MMS for healthy people**	191
14	**MMS for animals**	194
15	**Vitamin C and other antioxidants**	197
16	**Further information on MMS**	201
17	**Legal aspects**	204
18	**Guidelines for healthy living**	207

18.1	Living consciously: thoughts and emotions	210
18.2	Living consciously: the physical body	220
18.3	Physical health checklist	221
18.3.1	Living consciously: fresh air	222
18.3.2	Living consciously: water and salt	222
18.3.3	Living consciously: food	224
18.3.4	Living consciously: your energy	234
18.3.5	Living consciously: cosmetics, shoes and clothing	238
18.3.6	Living consciously: your home and workplace	246
18.3.7	Living consciously: vaccinations	249
19	**Your health in your hands**	**256**

About the author 260

Appendix
Directory of health practitioners and advisors with experience of MMS 262
Index 270

Foreword by Jim Humble

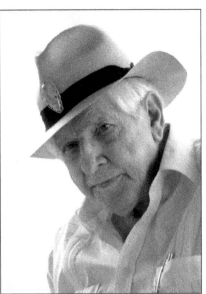
Photo: Adam Abraham

I came to Germany to give a week-long MMS training seminar in Fulda. Dr Antje Oswald and Leo Koehof picked me up from the airport.

While Dr Antje Oswald was working on the book you are now holding, we were in contact frequently to discuss the project. Now we were meeting for the concluding discussion. We discussed the newest MMS protocols, including the most current updates. We sat together for two days and went through The MMS Handbook *in its entirety. We talked about what I had discovered and about her experiences over 25 years of medical and homeopathic practice. I am inspired by her profound understanding of health and illness.*

I also find her self-conception as a doctor inspiring: she is convinced that everybody possesses the capacity for self-healing that will allow them to become well once they have identified and addressed the root cause of an illness. The information necessary to achieve this is clearly explained in this book.

At the same time she emphasises your personal responsibility for your own health.

In my opinion you will find that the necessary principles for gaining or maintaining good health are brilliantly set out here. In addition, The MMS Handbook *contains all the important, up-to-date information on MMS you need.*

I am delighted that the book is now finished and is to be published for all the world to read. All the best!

Jim Humble
October 2010

Foreword to the expanded Edition

The first edition of *The MMS Handbook* was out of print within two months, with the result that the second edition was published unchanged. Many thanks to all the readers for the interest you have shown. Continuing demand has now made a third and further editions possible.

New findings have induced me to revise *The MMS Handbook* and to make additions on a few matters, for example chlorine dioxide solution (CDS), slow activation based on the Fischer method, the addition of sodium bicarbonate for taste improvement and neutralisation, MMS eye drops, and much more.

Thanks are due to all who have shared their experiences with me, especially Dr Emmanuel Akuamoa-Boateng and his wife Gudrun Akuamoa-Boateng, Ali Erhan, Gerhard Feustle, Dr Hartmut Fischer, Dr Andreas Kalcker, Leo Koehof, Lothar Paulus, Dr Wolfgang Storch and, of course, Jim Humble.

Antje Oswald M.D.

Introduction

I did not seek out MMS, it found me. I first heard of it in 2009 when I attended a seminar at the Heilakademie Bauer. I ordered Jim Humble's book, *Breakthrough: The Miracle Mineral Supplement of the 21st Century*, immediately and read it in three days because I was so fascinated by the effectiveness of MMS. It seemed like a miracle to me. If all this is true, I thought to myself, MMS will be of invaluable help to mankind. Such potential. If everything Jim Humble writes here proves to be true, MMS can cure illnesses deemed incurable, can free Africa and Asia from tropical illnesses, can revolutionise our health system, because we will no longer need expensive antibiotics, no chemotherapy, no vaccinations, and there will be no need to fear infections … a wonderful prospect.

But how could I be sure that it worked? I decided to experiment on myself. At the next opportunity, I abstained from taking homeopathic remedies and gave a looming bout of sinusitis three days to develop. I then used MMS. It worked quickly. Within a few minutes a funny crackling noise in the maxillary sinuses indicated that something was happening. I felt better after taking the second dose. That impressed me and prompted me to experiment further on myself. Of course, I felt sick and had diarrhoea. That can happen when you attempt to determine where the tolerance threshold lies. It passes.

The experiment was worth it.

I now knew that what Jim Humble claimed regarding MMS was true, insofar as I could verify it on myself.

I consequently wrote a book review for *Homöopathie-aktuell*, the quarterly journal of the German Society for the Promotion of Natural Healing (Deutsche Gesellschaft zur Förderung naturgesetzlichen Heilens e.V.). Although MMS has nothing to do with homeopathy, I believed that it could be of interest to homeopaths and patients who prefer homeopathy to know that there is a remedy that fights pathogens effectively and expels heavy metal toxicity from the human body without evidence of damage to healthy cells. Things began to take their course. The publisher Daniel Peter called me in February 2010 and asked me whether I would be interested in writing my own book about MMS. I am glad I accepted his offer. And I am delighted that accepting his offer meant

Introduction

that I had the opportunity to meet Jim Humble on numerous occasions. Like most people who meet him personally, I am very fond of his quiet, humorous and affectionate way.

Since then I have come to know many people who have had moving experiences as a result of using MMS, either because they have been cured themselves, or because they have observed others being cured by it. Whereas previously I believed that MMS could be useful, I now know that it is. If you would like to know whether MMS could help you, just keep reading.

The book you are holding contains all the information you need. Only you can decide whether or not to go ahead and experiment. No one else can decide for you because little else is as important as the experiences you have as a result of making a decision to take responsibility for your own well-being.

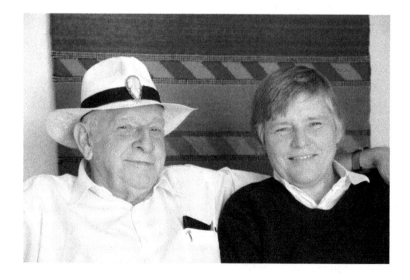

1

HOW IT ALL BEGAN

Once upon a time there was a brave man called Jim Humble who set out into the rainforest prospecting for gold. He returned without gold but with a treasure that was much more valuable than he could ever have dreamed of.

What sounds like the beginning of a fairy tale continues as an exciting crime thriller – and it is still unclear how the story will end. Who is Jim Humble and what drove him, at the age of 64, to undertake a jungle expedition in Inner Guyana instead of enjoying his retirement years? After all, he had already experienced adventures in plentiful supply.

Jim Humble is sitting comfortably in his apartment in Las Vegas, Nevada, when the telephone rings. An old friend from Chicago wants to know whether or not he would be interested in taking part in a gold mining project in the jungles of South America. Jim Humble is well known for the special gold mining techniques he has developed and which protect both the environment and the health of the workers; he is also well known for his ability to locate gold in the first place. The details are taken care of quickly. Jim Humble needs one month for the preparations. He sends his equipment on ahead. As part of his own personal provision he packs a number of bottles of stabilised oxygen so that he is able to use natural water resources as drinking-water. He once contracted typhus after drinking river water in the jungle and it is an experience he wants to avoid repeating.

Humble had heard from various sources that stabilised oxygen kills pathogens, especially if left in water over a long period of time. To be on the safe side, he tests this by adding stabilised oxygen to sewage water and has it analysed in a laboratory. The results show that all pathogens have been killed.

As a result, Jim Humble is confident that he will be able to obtain sterile water even when cut off from civilization, deep in the rainforest.

During the summer of 1996, he arrives at the airport in Georgetown. This city of about 33,000 residents is the capital of Guyana, a small state on the northern coast of South America. The country is sparsely populated, with most people living on the coast. Due to its proximity to the equator, unfavourable climate conditions prevail in the tropical rainforest in the interior of the country.

One of the contractual partners is related to Moses Nagamoto, Guyana's First Minister, and as a result Jim Humble is invited to dinner with the First Minister on the second day after his arrival. During their conversation Humble learns that Mr Nagamoto suffers from back pains so Humble, who has chiropractic training, offers to treat him. The pains soon abate. The following day, Humble is invited back, this time to treat the minister's daughter. The result is another satisfied patient. In this way, Jim Humble quickly gains an influential friend. Through him he comes to know other people from the government's most powerful circles such as the Minister of Mines, Jim Punwasee, who shows Humble the government's gold laboratory. A number of employees had been complaining that extremely poisonous mercury vapour was escaping through the ventilation system into the government building's courtyard and from there making its way back into the building. When Jim Humble suggests designing a simple, improvised air scrubber made out of a sprayer, two barrels and a few thousand table-tennis balls – which, as it turns out, works well – the government officials are delighted. To have made so many friends before setting out would stand Humble in good stead later.

He begins his jungle expedition, together with the landowner Mike and eight porters; other contractual partners and participants will join them later.

The long, arduous journey into the interior is undertaken partly in lorries and partly on boats. After crossing the river at Bortica, their entire luggage is loaded onto two lorries whose wheels have a diameter of two meters. Wheels of this size are necessary because the ground in the jungle is marshy and even so-called roads are in poor condition. Most of the porters prefer to take a short cut by foot because the lorries make such slow progress on the swampy roads and to avoid having to concentrate on not being thrown off the lorry on the bumpy journey. After travelling for five hours, everyone falls asleep wherever they can find a spot, somewhere outside. In the mornings the entire equipment is loaded onto boats. They head upriver along the Cuyuni arm. After travelling for four hours, the porters haul the entire luggage for the last part of the stage. They load everything onto their heads and backs, and fasten them with straps so that the main load rests on the head. This way each porter is able to carry up to 36kg. They face a two-day march through the rainforest with humidity levels of 100–110%. When, after a few days, two of his men fall ill with malaria, Jim Humble finds himself in a precarious situation. He has not taken any precautions against this eventuality because he had been told that malaria is not a problem in this part of Guyana. It is impossible for him to fetch help quickly because the region is so remote. He is unable to use the radio or telephone to call for help since radio equipment only works over short distances and there are no mobile telephone networks available. He decides to send two men to the nearest mine; it will be two to six days before they return. The patients are in a bad state. They lie there feverish and shivering, suffering from nausea, diarrhoea, headaches, and painful joints and muscles.

Jim Humble is determined to help them and comes up with the idea of giving the two sick men stabilised oxygen. He knows that this substance kills pathogens in water and that the human body is made up of over 70% water. The good news is that he has some in his luggage.

The two men agree to try the stabilised oxygen and Humble gives them a generous dose in some water. After only four hours the two men feel considerably better, so much so that they can even stand up. When on the following day two other men fall ill with malaria, they too are given stabilised oxygen and are well again by the afternoon. In only a short space of time, all the men are fit and well and able to work once more. Jim Humble is ecstatic.

In the period that follows, Humble gives all the malaria patients he meets stabilised oxygen and achieves a success rate of about 70%. One resident, suffering from malaria and typhus and in a very poor condition, reported significant improvements within only a few hours. Spurred on by this success and inspired by the desire to help malaria sufferers, Jim Humble decides to sell stabilised oxygen in Guyana. When he arrives back in Georgetown he places advertisements announcing this news, and it quickly spreads via newspapers, radio and TV. He is besieged by reporters. Within a few days he is famous. However, a few days later, the Guyanese Health Minister prohibits further sales of the solution, under punishment of imprisonment.

Humble later learns that two pharmaceutical companies had requested the Health Minister to forbid him to sell the solution, or they would otherwise no longer supply the local hospital with medication. Jim Humble continues to sell stabilised oxygen to those who need it and, as a result, charges are brought against him. He flees into the jungle, knowing that the residents of Georgetown – including the police – are so afraid of the wilderness that they are unlikely to follow in pursuit. Room for manoeuvre is afforded him as a result of his good relationship with government officials. He actually finds a productive gold-mine. Hitherto he has financed a large part of the enterprise from his own pocket. When Joel K., one of the principal shareholders in the venture, finally arrives and sees that the mine is yielding gold, he wants to claim most of the profits for himself and offers Jim Humble a 3% profit share instead of the 20% he had previously promised. When Jim Humble refuses to agree to this, Joel K. has the whole structure torn down because he is only liable to pay a profit share if he uses Humble's methods. As a result, it is pointless for Humble to remain in the jungle any longer.

Six months later the commotion surrounding the 'malaria solution' had abated. His friends in government circles had put in a good word for him. Jim Humble is now free to travel back to the USA. He is no longer interested in gold. He is now rather more interested in the composition of stabilised oxygen and in the reasons why it is sometimes effective against malaria, and sometimes not.

A few months later Jim Humble flies to Guyana once more. Another gold mining company has requested permission to use his gold mining techniques. When Humble himself becomes ill with malaria, he asks to be transported to the hospital in Georgetown for a blood test. Even though he is very ill and the journey back to civilization is difficult, he waits before taking his 'malaria solution' so that the hospital can first carry out a blood test. It conclusively proves that he has malaria. He takes his own 'medicine' and feels considerably better after only a few hours.

He has his blood tested again in order to complete the body of evidence. The results come back negative; the malaria can no longer be detected.

Jim Humble is now completely convinced that he has found a 'miracle medicine'. He decides to carry out further research on the substance and to make the results known throughout the world.

THE STUDY AND DISCOVERY OF MMS

In his endeavour to discover what stabilised oxygen is, what it is composed of, and how it acts, Jim Humble studies how oxygen is used in the human body. He comes to the realisation that the oxygen present in stabilised oxygen does not kill pathogens.

So what does kill the malaria parasites? The producers of stabilised oxygen keep their formula a commercial secret.

Jim Humble performs some experiments of his own. The usage instructions provided by one company state that stabilised oxygen should not be left standing for more than an hour because it breaks down in water. Curious, Humble puts ten drops in about 230ml of water and allows it to stand for ten hours. When he returns, he smells an odour similar to chlorine. Over the course of a series of experiments he uses thousands of test strips and various chemicals. In doing so he establishes that water lowers the alkaline value of the stabilised oxygen, that is, it causes it to become more neutral. In further tests, he adds acetic acid to cause the alkaline value of the stabilised oxygen to decrease further. By doing this, and by allowing the solution to stand for longer periods of time (24 hours), the chlorine odour becomes more and more discernible. Now at last he knows he is onto something. He obtains chlorine test strips from swimming pool suppliers. He waits patiently, observes, and repeats the procedure over and over again.

He finds the solution to the problem in 1998. He discovers that sodium chlorite is the effective agent – although at that time he still did not know what the active component was – and finds out over the course of further experiments that the addition of a 5% acetic acid solution considerably increases its effectiveness and that the solution reaches its full effect after only three minutes. While using only stabilised oxygen in water did not prove effective for all malaria patients (about 70%), the use of stabilised oxygen activated with a 5% acetic acid solution achieved a 100% success rate. Jim Humble's friends in Africa, whom he had been keeping up to date with the results of his experiments,

Sodium chlorite solution

report back to him the same results. He promptly receives positive feedback, some of which is included in his book *Breakthrough: The Miracle Mineral Supplement of the 21st Century*.

Sodium chlorite solution is alkaline. When acid is added to it, the OH-ions produced by the hydrolysis reaction are neutralised. The sodium hydroxide, which is a minor component in the solution, is also neutralised. Due to the influence of surplus acid, chlorine dioxide is formed from the chlorous acid ($HClO_2$) that is released from the oxidisation of ClO_2 ions, as shown in the equation below:

$$HClO_2 + HClO_3 \rightleftarrows 2ClO_2 + H_2O$$

The pure, gaseous chlorine dioxide has a yellow tinge to it and smells like chlorine. Chlorine dioxide is made up of one chlorine and two oxygen atoms. Chlorine dioxide is a hazardous substance, reacts oxidatively, has a tendency to decompose explosively, and cannot easily be stored because it corrodes all container materials. When it is required, it is produced on location for immediate use. It exercises specific oxidative effects against pathogens which kill the disease-causing organisms.

One website selling chlorine dioxide disinfectants presents the following abridged list of bacteria, viruses and fungi that chlorine dioxide kills. (Source: www.chlordioxid-academic.com)

Chlorine dioxide's spectrum of effectiveness

Adenovirus
Adenovirus echovirus
Aspergillus
Aspergillus flavus
Aspergillus niger
Bacillus
Bacillus cereus
Bacillus circulans
Bacillus megatarium
Bacillus subtilis
Bifidobacterium liberium
Bluetongue virus
Campylobacter jejuni
Candida
Candida albicans
Clostridium
Clostridium difficile
Clostridium perfringens
Clostridium sporogenes
Coliforms
Corynebacterium nucleatum
Coxsackievirus
Culex quinquefasciatus
E. coli
Echovirus
Encephalomyocarditis virus
Enterobacter cloacae
Enterobacter hafnia

Enterococcus faecalis
Feline parvovirus
Flavobacterium species
Fonsecaea pedrosoi
Fusarium species
Fusobacterium nucleatum
Human herpes virus I
Human herpes virus II
Influenza
Iridovirus (PPA)
Klebsiella
Klebsiella pneumoniae
Minute Virus of Mice (MVM)
Mouse encephalomyelitis virus
Mouse flu
Mouse Hepatitis Virus (MHV)
Mouse poliovirus
Mucor species mycobacterium
Mycobacterium kansasii
Mycobacterium smegmatis
Mycoplasma
Newcastle Disease Virus
Parainfluenza
Penicillium
Pertiviries-togaviridae
Poliovirus

Proteus vulgaris
Pseudomonas
Pseudomonas aeruginosa
Pseudomonas species
Saccharomyces cerevisiae
Salmonella
Salmonella choleraesuis
Salmonella gallinarum
Salmonella typhimurium
Salmonella typhosa
Sarcina lutea
Scopulariopsis species
Staphylococcus
Staphylococcus aureus
Staphylococcus epidermis
Stomatitis
Streptococcus
Streptococcus faecalis
Streptococcus pyogenes
Trichophyton
Trichophyton mentagrophytes
Trichophyton rubrum
Tuberculosis
Vaccinia virus
Vesicular stomatitis virus
Vibrio cholerae
Yersinia enterocolitica

The number of pathogens – some of which are particularly tenacious – that can be oxidised with chlorine dioxide is substantial. Moreover, I am not aware of any pathogenic bacterium or virus that cannot be oxidised using chlorine dioxide. When a pathogen comes into contact with chlorine dioxide, it decays and can no longer harm.

All that remains for the body to do is to manage the excretion of the dead pathogen. The chlorine dioxide is reduced by taking on electrons. The central atom thereby changes from oxidation state +4 to +/-0 or to the lowest possible of -1 as a chloride ion. Various reaction products may form as a result, depending on the conditions.

Oxygen ions are neutral; they join together with hydrogen to form water as a result of the decay of the chlorine dioxide during the oxidisation process.

> To summarise: when pathogens are killed by using dissolved chlorine dioxide, those pathogens decay and become harmless, as does the oxidising agent chlorine dioxide, which transforms into salt and water.

Reaction products: salt / water

After further tests and experiments, Jim Humble decides to produce a solution which he initially calls the 'Miracle Mineral Supplement'. He has since changed its name to 'Master Mineral Solution'. It is the same solution; only the name has changed. For simplicity's sake we will call it MMS, the name by which it became well known. This new formulation consists of a 28% solution of 80% technical grade sodium chlorite ($NaClO_2$). The other 20% of the salt is made up of excipients normally used to produce and stabilise sodium chlorite powder. That is about 19% sodium chloride (NaCl = cooking salt), and about 1% sodium hydroxide (NaOH) and sodium chlorate ($NaClO_3$). The actual sodium chlorite content is only 22.4% and is therefore about seven times stronger than in stabilised oxygen, which normally contains 3.5% sodium chlorite. By adding acid, such as vinegar, the alkaline sodium chlorite solution becomes slightly acidic, thereby becoming unstable, and releases chlorine dioxide as a result. Chlorine dioxide, like chlorine, has been used to purify water for over 100 years; it is also used in hospitals as a disinfectant. The US Food and Drug Administration agency has approved chlorine dioxide for use as a food steriliser. Chlorine dioxide is also

Master Mineral Solution

Sodium chlorite (NaClO2), not to be confused with sodium chloride (NaCl), cooking salt

Chlorine dioxide

used in Europe as a water purifier. It is safer and healthier to use chlorine dioxide as a water purifier than it is to use chlorine for the same purpose. At least three carcinogenic compounds form in drinking-water that contains chlorine. As we have already seen, salt and water are the only residual substances left behind by chlorine dioxide.

Some rich countries such as Saudi Arabia choose to use chlorine dioxide rather than chlorine to purify their drinking-water because it effectively kills pathogens and because it is harmless to human health in the quantities used. Since chlorine dioxide is significantly more expensive, poorer countries or municipalities fall back on chlorine, accepting that the drinking-water supplied contains carcinogenic compounds.

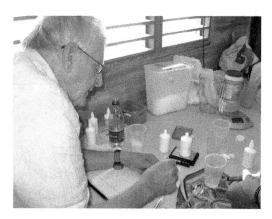

That will only change when enough people become aware of the influence the quality of the water they drink has on their health, and insist on having an adequate supply of good quality drinking-water.

Chlorine dioxide is the substance that kills germs, the substance Jim Humble spent almost two years searching for. Now he has found it. What baffled him is that no one before him had thought of testing the effect of chlorine dioxide on humans. Its ability to kill pathogens had, after all, been long known. And so he began to wonder whether it could possibly be against the pharmaceutical industry's interests to have a preparation on the market that could be used against all infectious diseases, a preparation that is reliable, that works – as far as we know – without any side effects, and that is extremely cheap in comparison to pharmaceutical drugs.

Even though Jim Humble made inquiries at a number of pharmaceutical companies, they refused to even test stabilised oxygen.

So Jim Humble undertook further investigations on his own.

Mode of action

Sodium chlorite ($NaClO_2$), in its pure state, is a white, crystalline salt that is fairly stable under normal conditions. It has a tendency to break down when the temperature rises sharply and a tendency to decay explosively when shaken, and when it is in contact with oxidable substances.

Sodium chlorite

To improve handling safety, the technical grade product that is produced commercially on a large scale contains 10 to 15% water, a small percentage of sodium chloride, depending on the process, and some sodium hydroxide (1%).

Sodium chlorite dissolves easily in water, and succumbs to hydrolysis in the water solution:

$$NaClO_2 + H_2O \rightleftharpoons Na^+ + OH^- + H^+ + ClO_2^-$$

By the term hydrolysis, we mean the breakdown of a salt by water, and the yielding of the acid and the alkaline from which the salt is formed.

Hydrolysis

Since $NaClO_2$ is the salt of a strong alkaline (NaOH) and a weak acid ($HClO_2$), the water solution reaction is alkaline overall because part of the chlorous acid formed is in balance with undissociated parts of the chlorous acid as shown in the equation:

$$H^+ + ClO_2^- \rightleftharpoons HClO_2$$

and because this lowers the concentration of H^+ ions. (In the presence of equally strong alkaline and acids, the water solution's reaction is neutral.)

When acids are added to the water solution of sodium chlorite, the dissociation balance of the above equation is moved in the direction of stronger dissociation of the chlorous acid. Because the chlorous acid is unstable, it breaks down further into chlorine dioxide (ClO_2). In addition, sodium chlorite forms chlorine dioxide when it comes into contact with hydrochloric acid as shown in this formula:

$$5\ NaClO_2 + 4\ HCl \rightarrow 5\ NaCl + 4\ ClO_2 + 2\ H_2O$$

3 • Mode of action

At temperatures of between -59°C and 11°C chlorine dioxide is an oily, amber liquid which is unstable and has a tendency to explode when the temperature rises above -40°C. At room temperature, chlorine dioxide is a gas. Solutions in water are yellow-brown and are not explosive as long as they do not produce a chlorine dioxide gas–air mixture with a chlorine dioxide ratio that is higher than 10% volume. Because of its volatility and high reactivity, it is produced on location for immediate or imminent use.

Production process for the preparation of drinking-water

As a result of Article 11 of the German Drinking Water Ordinance of 2009, the following production processes are standard in Germany:

The chlorine-chlorite process

$$2\ NaClO_2 + Cl_2 \rightarrow 2\ ClO_2 + 2\ NaCl$$

and the

Hydrochloric acid-chlorite process

$$5\ NaClO_2 + 4\ HCl \rightarrow 4\ ClO_2 + 5\ NaCl + 2\ H_2O.$$

A production process using sodium peroxide sulphate was approved in 2009: $2NaClO_2 + Na_2S_2O_8 \rightarrow 2\ ClO_2 + 2\ Na_2SO_4$

In Germany, the defined limit of chlorite (ClO_2^-) that drinking-water may contain after disinfection is 0.2mg ClO_2/litre; in exceptional cases 0.4mg/litre is allowed.

The toxicological review of chlorine dioxide and chlorite by the EPA (US Environmental Protection Agency) in Washington D.C. reported in September 2000 that higher organisms are relatively insensitive to the oral intake of chlorine dioxide. In one study on humans, no adverse changes were observed in ten healthy men when they swallowed a single dose of 24mg of chlorine dioxide in a litre of water, or 2.5mg of chlorite in 500ml of water. There were no negative results despite taking 10 to 100 times more than that allowed by the German Drinking Water Ordinance.
(Source: http://de.wikipedia.org/wiki/Chlordioxid, accessed 21/11/2010)

From that we can conclude with a probability bordering on certainty, that the dose recommended by Jim Humble for internal use is safe.

It has been proven that chlorine dioxide, as an oxidiser, kills pathogens very effectively. It can even kill bacteria that are resistant to antibiotics. This is because chlorine dioxide has a different mode of action from an antibiotic. It makes no difference to chlorine dioxide whether the pathogen concerned is susceptible to antibiotics or not. They are oxidised either way. However, chlorine dioxide is neither toxic to cells nor does it form free radicals.

Bacteria cannot develop resistance to chlorine dioxide

> Thomas Lee Hesselink explains in detail what scientists know about the oxidative effect of chlorine dioxide.
> (Source: Jim Humble, *Breakthrough*, Fourth Edition, Chapter 23)

I have summarised the main points here:

Summary

1. Oxidising agents cause living red blood cells to release more oxygen into the tissue. In turn, oxygen under elevated pressure is a powerful detoxifier of carbon monoxide, supports the natural healing processes of the body in cases of burns, crush injuries, and ischaemic strokes, and is effective against bacterial infections.
2. Many oxidising agents are effective in stimulating the immune system when taken internally on a regular basis. White blood cells are induced to produce cytokines. These in turn function in the body as an alarm system, induce cells to attack pathogens, and prevent allergic reactions. Activated cells of the immune system produce, as part of the inflammatory process, natural oxidising agents such as hydrogen peroxide (H_2O_2), peroxynitrate (-OONO) and hypochlorous acid (HOCl). These work by eliminating pathogens or cancerous cells.
3. A variety of oxidising agents, chlorine dioxide in particular, are used worldwide for disinfection purposes because their bacteriostatic or bactericidal and virucidal function has long been known. In the extensive list of sources included in this article, you will find materials on the use of chlorine dioxide to eliminate various bacteria and viruses, including hepatitis, HIV and polioviruses. There are also many studies that prove that the malaria pathogens Plasmodium vivax, Plasmodium falciparum, Plasmodium ovale and Plasmodium malariae are sensitive to oxidising agents such as chlorine dioxide.

Oxidising agent

The ability of Plasmodia to live and grow – as with bacteria and cancer cells – is dependent on there being an abundance of thiol compounds. When thiols react with chlorine dioxide, which they do very easily, it forms disulphide (RSSR), disulphide monoxide (RSSOR), sulphenic acid (RSOH), sulphinic acid (RSO_2H), and sulphonic acid (RSO_3H), all of which destroy the life processes of Plasmodia. If the chlorine dioxide destroys enough thiols, the parasite dies. Moreover, the chlorine dioxide lowers the quantity of reduced glutathiones available to the parasites; they need the glutathione for their detoxification processes to avoid poisoning themselves when digesting the protein from the haemoglobin of red blood cells and the metabolic products that result from the process. This is because each digested haemoglobin molecule releases four heme molecules as a by-product. These molecules are redox active, react with the surrounding oxygen, and in doing so produce oxygen peroxide and other toxic oxidising agents that poison the parasites internally. This is why Plasmodia must constantly and quickly eliminate heme molecules, which can only be done with reduced glutathione. Because sodium chlorite and chlorine dioxide oxidise glutathione they bring about the destruction of the malaria pathogen. A number of common malaria medicines such as quinine, chloroquine, and mefloquine work by blocking the heme elimination process.

Over time, a number of malaria pathogens have developed resistance through increased production of glutathione. This can be reversed with chlorine dioxide because just one chlorine dioxide molecule oxidises five glutathione molecules, thereby making them harmless.

4. Polyamines are vital for the survival of tumours, bacteria and parasites. If they are unavailable, the pathogen dies, and tumour cells can no longer grow and will also die. It is known that chlorine dioxide destroys polyamines through oxidisation.

You will find further scientific studies on oxidation and reduction processes on the internet at:

www.bioredox.mysite.com

The effect of internal administration of chlorine dioxide on blood condition is striking. This dark-field microscope image demonstrates how a blood clot has been dissolved within an hour of drinking chlorine dioxide in water. Moreover, the blood cells appear to be well-rounded and healthier.

Mode of action

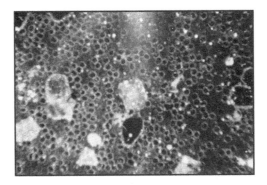

Blood sample from a male test subject

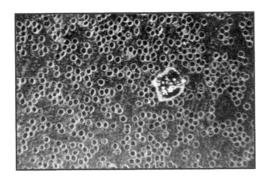

Blood sample from the same male test subject about 1 hour later

The dark-field microscope images were taken by Martina Schmidt, a specialist advisor on health management at the Chemnitz Harmony Trade Fair 'Health for Body, Mind and Spirit'; they were made available by Dr Wolfgang Storch. The same improvement in the structure of the blood was reproduced with a female test subject, and a similar result achieved even when the time between taking the dose and taking the photograph was reduced to only 20 minutes.

Erythrocytes react with chlorine dioxide in just as specific a way as they do with oxygen. In the concentration and dosage recommended by Jim Humble, the MMS solution, mixed with the acid and diluted with water, releases chlorine dioxide in the body for at least an hour. Since the erythrocytes do not distinguish between oxygen and chlorine dioxide, they transport chlorine dioxide in the blood just as they do oxygen, to wherever the body needs oxygen. They then release chlorine dioxide there. Pathogens cannot survive in the presence of chlorine dioxide because of the oxidation process. Although chlorine dioxide has at least 100 times more

Erythrocytes transport chlorine dioxide to the seat of the disease

energy than oxygen, it does not harm healthy cells, or healthy bacterial flora. To put it more precisely, it has not been observed that chlorine dioxide reacts with healthy cells in the concentration and dosage used by Jim Humble. He suspects that this is due to the fact that healthy cells are better able to hold on to their electrons because they are used for oxidative processes. As a result, they cannot be oxidised as easily as the more unstable pathogenic agents and acidic elements.

Chlorine dioxide not only kills pathogens, it can also neutralise toxins. Because most substances harmful to humans are acidic, chlorine dioxide has a detoxifying effect when it encounters acidic substances.

Metals are oxidised   Are there any findings which explain why it is effective against heavy metals? Metals are easily oxidised. Consider iron that is exposed to air – a wrought-iron gate, for example. If it is not treated in a certain way – by galvanization, for instance – it will gradually rust. Rust is formed as a decomposition product following the oxidisation of iron. It is not as firm or as stable as iron itself and can easily be removed. It is in the nature of metals to become oxidised, and it is in the nature of chlorine dioxide to oxidise. After oxidisation, the metals have lost their stability and can be eliminated by the body.

The immune system is supported   If the chlorine dioxide encounters neither pathogens nor acidic substances in the body, according to Jim Humble it will slowly decompose. In doing so, it will grab one or two electrons at most. An intermediate product is thereby produced, from which the body produces hypochlorous acid, one of the supporting pillars of the immune system. The human organism needs hypochlorous acid to eliminate pathogens and even cancer cells. Chlorine dioxide can, therefore, support the human organism in one way or another in patients with any disease that requires an immune response from the body, and it appears it can do so extremely effectively.

Convincing results   The above section is based on information made available by Jim Humble, based on his extensive research and experiments. Naturally, as a single individual he was only able to work within certain limits. No claim to scientism in the sense common today is made. However, the results speak for themselves and are more than enough to convince most users.

It would be valuable to conduct further research on the effect of chlorine dioxide on the human biosystem. The only question is: who would be willing to pay for it?

Such a research project demands highly-educated specialists, a few years, and a suitable research setting. This is because far more complex processes take place in the human body than occur in the field of inorganic chemistry, where certain reactions can be carried out and described in isolation.

Fortunately Andreas Kalcker, a biophysicist who lives in Spain, has become interested in this subject. He is working with MMS and chlorine dioxide within the university system. He surmises that the main effect of chlorine dioxide is based on physical phenomena, which is why it has a positive effect and such a wide range of indications. We can look forward with excitement to finding out his discoveries.

However, it is not absolutely necessary to know exactly how and why MMS works before making practical use of it. Incidentally, it is not always known how several pharmaceutical medicines work either. When experience shows that a substance is effective and does no harm, it is an excellent idea to make use of it, even if there is need for further research since not all aspects of its mode of action can yet be explained conclusively.

Certainly, Thomas Lee Hesselink concludes that the application of sodium chlorite as recommended by Jim Humble is very useful since the method is easy to use, inexpensive, and evidently completely nontoxic.

———————————————————————————————4

REMARKABLE THERAPEUTIC SUCCESSES

When the original edition of Jim Humble's book *Breakthrough: The Miracle Mineral Supplement of the 21st Century* was first published, he had already received numerous reports of malaria patients who had been cured.

The German translation, *MMS: Der Durchbruch* (published by Mobiwell Verlag), included some of the many letters that Jim Humble received, all reporting the swift cure experienced by many malaria sufferers who had been given his 'malaria solution'. One example is a letter from Ev. John Tumuhairwe, a pastor in Uganda, in which he reports that HIV-positive soldiers were successfully treated using Humble's 'malaria solution'.
(Source: Jim Humble, *Breakthrough: The Miracle Mineral Supplement of the 21st Century*, p. 74; ISBN 978-0-9792884-4-9)

Manfred Romann, a German who had been infected with malaria when he was a prisoner of war in the Russian marshland of the Volga and who had suffered ever since, has also recovered using MMS (see Experience Report 'Malaria', pp. 78–9).

Film: Under- In the film *Understanding MMS* (by Daniel Peter Verlag), a number
standing of colleagues report how MMS helped their patients, or indeed how
MMS it cured them from illness. But first, heed Jim Humble's words in the film.

> Jim Humble: Over the past many months I have been talking to hundreds of people on the phone and have received thousands of emails and I'm coming to realise that the microorganisms in the body are affecting the body much more than people think – and much more than even the American Medical Association thinks. People come to us and take a few doses of MMS, and pains that they've had for twenty years disappear within an hour or two or three. I have had people walk in there with a cane, barely

able to walk, and two or three hours later they throw the cane away. And it's all because the microorganisms that have been sitting in there in various joints and muscles have been killed. When they're gone, the pain is gone, and the body is ready to start functioning at an improved level.

Diabetes

... this is Kino Bay, Mexico, and right near here is a small restaurant and the woman who owns the restaurant is a Mexican lady. I handed her a bottle of MMS one day when she had the flu and said: 'Here, take this.' I explained that she should activate it with lemon juice. I did not have a book to give her. I just told her to take it and she did. She had quite severe diabetes. She had to inject herself with insulin every day. After taking MMS for a couple of weeks she stopped injecting herself and she did not notice any of the symptoms of diabetes any more. I don't know whether she's going to a doctor about it or not, but she's not having to inject herself and she's feeling fine.

The American physician Dr John Humiston, who practiced in Tijuana, Mexico, at the time (and who is now in San Diego, California), talks in the film about MMS' spectrum of efficacy and mode of action:

Is MMS dangerous?

When it comes to medications and therapies, the first thing you look at is safety, the second thing is efficacy. Is it safe to take? That's always the most important thing. MMS in its prescribed doses – I don't think it could be dangerous for anybody. I have used it on all my children; they're ages 2 to 17. I think we were probably using it on our two-year-old before he was two.

Professor Antonio Romo Paz, a chemist at the University of Sonora, Mexico, describes his experiences with MMS.

My name is Antonio Romo Paz and I'm a chemist. I'm a professor at the University of Sonora. I found out about this product from Clara Beltrones and I was immediately interested in it. I had already heard of it at some seminars on products that strengthened the immune system at the University of Mexico. My interest was instantly aroused when she said that it regulates the immune system. I then began to do some research to find out more about MMS, or chlorine dioxide. I searched through the bibli-

Laryngitis

ography and I became more and more interested because MMS regulates the immune system. I then took it myself because I had a cold and laryngitis and I felt better instantly. I felt completely well on the following day. So I continued to use this chlorine dioxide, this strong oxidising substance, and recommended it to others, persuaded friends to take it. A friend of mine, a forty-year-old woman, suffered from intestinal parasites known as giardia.

Intestinal parasites

I had come across this parasite through my work so I was familiar with it. I knew that chlorine dioxide was very effective but it had never been tested on humans. I decided to use Jim Humble's method, adding a few drops of citric acid to chlorine dioxide, and to give the person who had tested positive to the parasites, to this amoeba, a dose of six drops twice daily for four days. We would conduct a further analysis after the four days. The woman tested negative and was very pleased. The standard treatment involves using Metronidazole, a carcinogenic substance which has a number of side effects. That medication is approved by the US Food and Drug Administration and people who take it suffer from intense trembling. Some even have convulsions. I advised my friend against taking it and instead recommended she take the chlorine dioxide with a few drops of citric acid added – the test results on the fourth day were negative. She felt well. She had intestinal colic and suffered bleeding but by the fourth day she was completely cured. I doubted these results because I had never seen such a thing before. I had thought that the dose would have to be increased but that wasn't necessary. Six drops twice a day for four days cured her of the parasite, a strong parasite, where the standard treatment would have involved severe side effects and would have attacked the stomach and the mucous membrane of the bowels.

Tuberculosis

… a number of the inmates of this prison (Author's note: Sonora State) suffer from tuberculosis. I recommended MMS to the medical staff here, encouraging them to try it out alongside the standard medication that they normally use. Being open-minded people, they agreed to try it out on the patients who did not respond well to the traditional medication that is used worldwide. They tried it on someone who was very resistant to every antibiotic … when a person turns out to be resistant, tuberculosis is very difficult to cure. He took the drops (Author's note: MMS drops) at a dose not all that high – only eight drops per day. We gave him the drops for a while, less than a month and then we carried out some tests that indicate whether or not the mycobacteria responsible for tuberculosis are still present. The results were negative. Everyone, including the doctors, was very surprised that this man was cured. Even though he continues to take the drops he is very happy and tells everyone that it was MMS that cured him.

Those are my experiences of MMS.

Genero Ignacio Argunio no longer suffers from psoriasis.

Psoriasis

I had psoriasis. Psoriasis is an incurable disease. It is hereditary. I had the plaque type of psoriasis. The areas of skin affected were inflamed, reddish, at the point of bleeding, and reached down into deeper skin layers. I was sent to see the doctor, who prescribed Cortisone, the only effective medication against such skin conditions. Antonio Romo Paz, a chemist and lecturer at the University of Sonora, recommended that I try MMS. He explained how to prepare it. It is sodium chlorite and by adding citric acid the chlorine produces free radicals that have an antiseptic, antibacterial effect on the skin. At that point my limbs, my ears (the ear cartilage), my elbows and knees were badly affected. But when I applied the MMS everything healed well. You can still see marks and scars, evidence of the illness is still visible, but it put an end to the psoriasis. It burned, it hurt so much I could have screamed, and it bled. But now it's over.

Later in the film, Adriana Cosme Duarte reports that her toothache, from which she had been suffering for four months, disappeared after she took MMS twice a day for four days. Jim Humble tells the story of a woman who was in the final stages of lung cancer (the doctors had told her she only had about two weeks to live). After eight days she was able to get out of bed and after eleven days she went for a walk and started to work again. Clara Beltrones reports that MMS cleared up her daughter's acute appendicitis and helped her mother who had a bad case of ischialgia. Dennis Richard tells us that his loose teeth became firm again after only a few days of brushing his teeth with MMS. Melvin Randolph, who had prostate cancer, reports that his PSA-levels were permanently reduced from 48.7 to 1.29 by using MMS.

Toothache

Lung cancer

Appendicitis

Ischialgia

Prostate cancer

These are some of the people who tell their stories with enthusiasm in the film *Understanding MMS*.

4 • Remarkable therapeutic successes

4.1 Experience reports from Belgium, Denmark, Germany, Great Britain, Austria, Switzerland and Mexico

The following MMS experience reports come from self-responsible users who have used MMS internally or externally with or without a doctor's supervision. Only a few were ready to publish their full names as they make the stories of their illness public. Therefore only initials are given in most cases. But I can assure you that behind each of these initials stands a real person who really experienced the exact story you are now reading. In some cases I have abridged the reports slightly, without changing the meaning or tone.

4.1.1 Experience reports from self-responsible users

09/12/2009: Ms S.

Pendunculated warts / age marks

Hello, been taking MMS 1 for a week and have started with one drop in the mornings and evenings. I'm now up to 5 drops – no side effects. Don't take it that regularly since I work shifts. Today I noticed that my pendunculated warts and my roughened age marks have disappeared. I'm excited to see what other changes will happen to my body.

10/12/2009: Ms I. Z., Switzerland

Intestinal Bacterium (ESBL)

A success story: the resistant intestinal bacterium ESBL cleared up using MMS 1. I (78 years old) was told about MMS 1 by some German friends. I had to undergo an operation on my intervertebral discs five years ago. Unfortunately I suffered damage to the nerves. I still have to take medication to this day just to retain any degree of mobility. MMS 1 has not helped in this regard yet. While in hospital, I contracted the intestinal bacterium ESBL, which is resistant to antibiotics and which, according to the doctors, cannot be eliminated. Over the course of the last five years I have had 34 bladder infections and have been given antibiotics 34 times. I first used MMS 1 in October 2009. After 14 days, the stool sample sent to the laboratory of infectiology was free from the ESBL bacterium – the result caused quite a stir at the laboratory – inexplicable. I still have problems with my bladder but it's 'free from bacteria'. I feel as if a huge burden has been taken away. Until now I could hardly take a holiday. I still need to address the other problem, the damage to the nerves in my intervertebral disc L 4/5. Is that possible? Maybe I should take MMS 2 as well? I'm very impressed with MMS 1 and am convinced of its effectiveness against various ailments.

01/09/2009: sent in for use in this book by Lothar Paulus

Report by Mr D. from Geislingen
I'd be happy for you to use my 'showcase' – but it is not the only one, I'll write this in telegram style:

- Boy, 6 years old, 22kg, asthma, treated with antibiotics for 3 years without success: after 1 week of MMS practically healthy, ice cream and cold cola without an attack for the first time in years. — *Asthma*
- Two girls, 6 years old, 18kg, after 1 week free from asthma.
- Man, about 70 years old, circulation problems on the right side of the body for a number of years, after one week (strong dose) nothing, could walk again, put on shoes without trouble. — *Circulation disorders*
- Woman, 70 years old, no eye specialist could help, no lens was strong enough. After 4 days she could read the instruction leaflet of a medication packet WITHOUT her glasses. And after a week no longer any problems climbing the stairs, felt 'new born'. — *Weak vision*
- Woman, 47 years old, inflamed haemorrhoids, gone after a week. — *Haemorrhoids*
- Girl, 18 years old, asthma since childhood, serious attacks, sometimes monthly, with emergency care at hospital. After 2 weeks on a low dose nothing, has been healthy ever since.
- And the best case is me myself, with a cyst the size of an egg on my back. Within two weeks it was gone. I simply can't explain it because a cyst is not an inflammation or anything similiar to one, but it's gone. — *Cysts*

14/12/2009: Ms S.

I have been taking MMS 1 for about six weeks. On the day I began to take 2 x 6 drops I no longer needed my asthma pump, which I'd needed twice a day previously. I could also throw away the support bandage on my right arm, which I had to use because of my arthritis, after two days. I bathe with MMS and my athlete's foot is disappearing gradually. The discharge I had has gone. I have recommended MMS to a friend, who is also completely — *Asthma* / *Athlete's foot* / *Arthritis* / *Discharge* won over by it. I'm flying to South Africa in January to see my children and I hope I can help many people there with it …

11/01/2010: Peter Schneider from Spalt

Chronic rhinitis

The case history almost sounds like a fairy tale, just not as amusing. Once upon a time in the year 1966 I broke my nasal bone in an accident at work. It wasn't too serious because it was only the septum (I thought). Over the years – I was in the German armed forces – I had breathing problems. One nostril always seemed to be constricted. They sent me to an ENT doctor, but he couldn't detect anything. And so I laboured on through life with a nose that became blocked more and more often. In 1985 it became so bad that I went to see the ENT doctor once more, because nasal sprays aren't too healthy when used long-term. But after various allergy tests – all negative – and examinations (the broken nose was not an issue) I was given a cream mixed by the doctor himself which was meant to regenerate the mucous membrane. It was a sweeping success – now I didn't get any air whatsoever. So I got rid of the cream and the doctor just like that. I went back to using nasal sprays – and have been doing so for the last 25 years. I always carried a spray bottle so that my voice didn't sound so 'French'. Now this is where it becomes interesting.

Sometime in 2009 I read about Jim Humble and his MMS in *Nexus* magazine. Since I'd always been a proponent of alternative medicine I bought the book and shortly thereafter ordered the MMS base and the citric acid as an activator. But I didn't even think of my nose at that point. I began with two drops, then on the next day I took four, then six, at which level I stayed for a week because that's what Jim recommends for people over 60. I did not observe any side effects and I felt well. A week later I must have caught a draught: nose blocked, itchy throat. Nip it in the bud, I thought – it was about midday when I allowed myself ten drops of MMS and at 4 p.m. I took another twelve drops. From 5.30 p.m. onwards I was free from complaints and stunned by the speed with which it took effect. I took another ten drops the next morning as a precaution. I hadn't noticed that I hadn't needed the nasal spray the whole day. In the evening, when I went to bed I was about to take the nasal spray to help me sleep but realised that my nose was still clear so I left it, but took the bottle with me to the bedroom. In the morning I could still breathe freely and I thought it was strange because I couldn't explain the reason for this sudden recovery.

In the meantime I have worked it out: it was the MMS. Martin Frischknecht speculated in one conversation we had whether it could have been heavy metal toxicity or a fungal infection. He is probably right and the MMS has done a good job of it. I'm sure I don't need to mention that I still take my six drops a day and have not had any complaints of any kind since. A number of family members and acquaintances have been cured of various minor ailments in no time. Anyone still going through life without MMS at their side only have themselves to blame!

12/10/2010: Peter Schneider again

Nail fungus

According to the statistics, one in five Germans has nail fungus. That's about sixteen million people. And I was one of them. It really is strange that the pharmaceutical industry can't come up with anything other than extremely expensive remedies such as nail polish, and medications whose side effects will sooner or later bring you close to a socially acceptable demise. (And why should they?) Thank goodness there's MMS 1. And now to yours truly:

Many years ago I had a couple of horses, one of whom trod on my left big toe. A few months after the injury had healed, I noticed a spot that had turned a yellowish colour and that a hollow had developed under the nail there. I went to the doctor and was given the usual remedies.

Were they successful? Not at all. This continued for a few years, and the affected area grew. I tried vinegar essence (a tip from a friend) with temporary success. The fungus did not develop. Unfortunately it started growing again a little later and nothing helped. I removed the hollow parts of the nail until only about a third of the nail remained. Something had to be done, if only from an aesthetic standpoint. By this time I was already familiar with MMS and had enjoyed my first successes with it. Having read about other uses of MMS in Jim's book, I began to experiment. Whatever helped internally against bacteria, viruses and fungi also had to work externally. I should say in advance that I'm a relatively rustic person when it comes to caring for my health, and what follows here should not necessarily be emulated.

I mixed two drops of MMS and after activating it I put it in a small syringe – undiluted. I then injected the solution under the remaining hollow parts in the nail. It's painless if you don't jab yourself. The whole nail bed became white and looked as if it had been whitewashed. I repeated this treatment daily for six weeks, removing the loose skin and nail parts after foot baths. I stopped the treatment after this period because I noticed that a new nail that wasn't hollow was growing from the nail root. Seven weeks have passed since then, the nail bed is a normal colour again and the nail is growing.

I hope it stays like that and that the nail grows back to its old size; that would be another victory for MMS.

Conclusion: you can certainly use MMS in unconventional ways. We know that no one has died of MMS – which can't be said of pharmaceuticals!

02/06/2010: Sophia P. from Bavaria reports on her family and her experiences with children.

Whooping cough
Eight-month-old infant, 7.5kg, had contact with two children infected with whooping cough. Three days later high fever (up to 39 °C), restlessness, cough setting in. Dose: 2 x 1 drop of MMS daily for five days. Within two hours of the first dose the fever breaks, gone twelve hours later. Cough improves on the first day, progress on the whole similar to having a slight cold.

Chickenpox
Eight-year-old girl with chickenpox, 28kg, fever for two days, severe, very itchy rash, restless and awake at night. Takes 1 x 2 drops of MMS, fever breaks after three hours, after five hours she can sleep. After taking a further dose of one drop of MMS the itchiness stops.

Bruises Cuts
Twelve-year-old boy, 45kg; falls on his face playing football. Bruises and cuts with severe swelling to the face. Takes 2 drops of MMS daily for three days. The severe swelling and the pains decrease within three days.

Infants and small children generally have good tolerance for and react well to MMS. There is a noticeable effect within a short time of taking the dose.

Ms Sophia P. continues.

Experience with adults:

Oedema
37-year-old woman in the ninth month of pregnancy with oedema in the legs, of medium severity. Simply by brushing her teeth with six drops of MMS for two days (3–4 times a day) the oedema clears up almost entirely.

68-year-old woman, 62kg, continued to have problems with sleep despite having taken sleeping tablets for decades. Since taking four drops of MMS at night and brushing her teeth with it, she has generally been consistently able to sleep.	*Sleep disorders*
By brushing teeth with MMS, some have experienced a reduction in sensitivity to cold and sweet foods.	*Sensitive teeth*

Sophia P. generally recommends:

> ... instead of the 6+6 protocol, that gives a total of 12 drops or even higher doses – unless absolutely necessary – it is preferable to take 4 × 3 = 12, spread over the day. By this I mean that it's better to take the same number of drops spread over the day but ensure that you stay within a 12-hour window so that the quantity takes effect simultaneously.

11/06/2010: Ms A. – success with Crohn's disease

Dear Sir, I waited a few extra days because a lot is going on here with MMS. The biggest success to report is, for me, that a friend of mine – she suffers from Crohn's disease, which is thought incurable – has been completely free of problems since following the MMS regimen. She'd been having infusions and taking Cortisone for months but these had mind-blowing side effects and did not help against the intestinal pains. She went back to her doctor after following the MMS regimen and was found to be free of the condition. Unfortunately, after a couple of weeks, her body started reacting again because she had dived back into the stress of everyday life. As soon as she took another small dose of six drops, the intestinal pains stopped. This demonstrates that it's important not just to address the symptoms but also to consider why the illness developed and what changes you need to make in your life. I'm still impressed nevertheless because Crohn's disease is considered incurable and MMS cleared up all symptoms within a week. I can personally testify to countless virus infections that I nipped in the bud with a single dose of 6 drops. If that does not clear it, then on taking another 6 drops an hour later everything is OK. Just one tip when taking it: I have tried it with various juices to mask the taste of chlorine. I tolerate banana juice best because juices that contain acid fail to mask the chlorine	*Crohn's disease*

taste fully. I started with the regimen myself two years ago. Up to 2 x 15 drops daily and then a week at that level. Some friends of mine had experienced a few 'miracle cures' after being on the regimen.

One no longer had hay fever, the other (a smoker) could breathe more easily. External application cleared up her warts and I was able to cure a badly inflamed insect bite on my foot after only one day.

24/06/2010: Britta E.

Fungal infection *Fibromyalgia*	MMS has helped young and old. I'd be delighted to tell you how MMS has helped me and my family. I had a fungal infection in the vaginal area. The appointment with the gynaecologist was in two days time. I took six drops of MMS before meals in the morning, at midday, and in the evening. When I went to see the doctor no fungal infection could be found. I would never have thought that MMS could be effective against fungal infections. Had fibromyalgia again with pains around the clock. Because I was still breastfeeding I couldn't take any medicines. I took MMS, after three days the pains were completely gone. Mobility improved by 60%. Now I'm on the second phase with 4 x 6 drops daily. I'll let you know.
Children: coughs and colds	I gave my two-year-old girl a bath with 15 drops when she coughed or sniffled. She was well again immediately afterwards. She also gets a drop of MMS and lemon with apple juice from time to time.
Swine flu	My daughter caught Swine flu from a school friend. She was given six drops of MMS immediately, and again after an hour, and once more before going to bed. She felt much better the next day. She continued to take six drops of MMS three times a day. She went back to school on the third day. Her school friend's battle against the illness continued, it took her three weeks to get better.
Toothaches	While being treated by the dentist I acquired a gum wound which became inflamed. It throbbed so badly at night that I could barely sleep a wink. I then saw Jim Humble's video where he explains that MMS is very effective for gums and he swears that the pains would be gone in an hour. I took 15 drops of MMS and gargled with it. After an hour I could confirm that his statement was true and I could finally sleep the whole night through undisturbed. The inflammation disappeared instantly.

A friend from Trossingen was diagnosed with inflammation of the gums. She would have to undertake a treatment costing 80 euros and made an appointment for two weeks later. During this time I advised her to take MMS, to gargle with it and to rub it in with a toothbrush. She took ten drops. Two weeks later the dentist, wide-eyed in wonder, could only establish that the inflammation was gone. He asked what she'd done but when she told him about MMS he just shook his head.	*Inflammation of the gums*
A friend's asthma cleared up. She'd never been able to breathe as deeply as she can since taking MMS. A winter without flu or asthma!	*Asthma*
A friend of mine had problems with digestion. She'd been unable to have a bowel movement for two weeks. I offered her some MMS. She only took six drops a day. On the following day she was able to pass a stool promptly and has been free of digestive problems ever since.	*Digestive problems*

July 2010: Nurhan B. from North Rhine-Westphalia treats nail fungus with MMS.

Dear Antje, my customers at the nail studio have benefited greatly from MMS. I applied a few drops of activated MMS mixed with some water onto the foot. Athlete's foot didn't have a chance. I have also had success with tough cases of nail fungus, if they take it externally at least three times daily and drink six drops twice a day.	*Nail fungus*
Baths (with 30 drops of MMS) have helped with psoriasis on the palms of the hands and on the soles of the feet, supplemented with six drops twice a day taken as a drink. I only have good things to say about MMS.	*Psoriasis*

07/07/2010: Johanna S. from Bielefeld has unobstructed respiratory passages once again.

I suffered from mucus obstruction of the airways for a long time: allergic rhinitis alternating with recurring sinusitis, sometimes in combination with bronchitis, made life hard. On 16/05/2010, I began with three drops of activated MMS daily because I had a bad infection of the upper air passages. Initially I reacted with an aggravated cough and hoarseness and I	*Allergic rhinitis alternating with recurring sinusitis*

sweated more and discharged yellow phlegm. The cough had more or less disappeared by the next day and my nose was unobstructed. On 18/05 I took four drops of MMS in the morning. Afterwards I was remarkably exhausted and slept for two hours in the afternoon, watery stool. On 19/05 I took another four drops of MMS in the afternoon, stool was normal again. It's had a great effect on the air passageways. I slowly increased to seven drops over the next few days. That agreed with me, phlegm discharge now and again. I took a break from 30/05 until 02/06 because I was sweating profusely and was coughing heavily as before 16/05. From 03/06 I started taking seven drops and slowly increased to 18 drops, which I have now been taking for ten days. I had skin reactions: small spots of puss on my face and a red patch on my calves. I feel well on the inside, I can breathe freely again, better than it's been for a long time.

Addendum on 26/10/2010: I'm very happy with the effect MMS has had, my airways are still clear.

20/07/2010: Udo B. (63 years old), Düsseldorf

Joint pains

Sleep disorders

We received the MMS on 29/06/2010. Without having read up much about it I took only one drop (1:1), out of curiosity, in the afternoon with a glass of water. I became tired and I slept for about 15 minutes. I woke up positively refreshed and the severe arthritic pains I'd had were as if they'd been 'blown away' in the truest sense of the word. I had been suffering from severe joint pains in both knees and elbows for over seven months. Because of the pains I had been afraid of going to lie down or of getting up from bed because when I did so the pains moved from the joints and into the limbs. And now, from one minute to the next, I was being freed – it was unbelievable. Over the following days I increased the dose to the current level of six drops.

I have had to take the neuroleptic 'Dipiperon, 40mg' every day for more than two years to treat insomnia and states of psychomotoric agitation. I have stopped taking it since starting on MMS. It has been a resounding success. I can finally sleep without after-effects during the day, light and refreshing, remarkably balanced, and am no longer gloomy during the day. A new freedom!

Experience reports

22/07/2010: Eva R., Altheim

My daughter (10 years old) had a wound of about 1.5cm long on her scalp for more than two years. It was a spot that she would often scratch when lost in thought. A scab would sometimes form on the wound; at other times it was scratched raw, and was partly inflamed. Hair no longer grew on this part. Then I came across MMS. I mixed the drops with the turbo activator and applied two drops, undiluted, directly onto the wound once a day. It burned slightly on the scalp and my daughter endured it without much fuss. I did that for about four or five days. The scab cleared and the wound had a clean edge. After about ten days the wound had healed and a nice thin layer of skin had formed. A short time afterwards my daughter scratched the area open again – probably out of habit. I applied the drops onto the wound once more and it closed without any problems – and a few days later you could see how the hair had begun to grow. There have been no problems since then and you can't even see a scar.

Itchy eczema on head

18/08/2010: sent by Stefan M., Bavaria

Ms M.'s ordeals began before Christmas 2007 when she started to suffer pains and prickling in her right foot; standing on it was painful. It was not easy for her, especially since she was responsible for a household that had two children of primary school age.

The pains became so bad in January 2008 that it became impossible to stand on the right foot, or to roll the foot from heel to toe. The pain intensified until it became unbearable. She had to go to hospital, and was admitted to a neurological ward.

She was diagnosed with an inflammation and paralysis of the sciatic nerve on the right side. She was unable to lift or lower her right foot. Various tests were made, such as a a lumbar puncture, MRT of the lower extremities, neurography scans, and EMG. The treatment involved taking strong painkillers (high doses of Gabapentin and Morphine) and antidepressants. Ms M. was discharged with '… reduced symptoms of pain with paraesthesia of the right foot as well as unsteady motion … '.

After further attempts at controlling the condition, including visits to various alternative practitioners, Ms M. was advised by the neurologist Dr K. to visit the neurology ward of the regional hospital because they had the equipment necessary to get to the bottom of her illness … So in August 2008 Ms M.

Sciatica

Depression

Vague soft tissue inflammation

Neurological symptoms

was admitted to the neurological department of the regional hospital, where further examinations were carried out, among them an MRT of the whole spine.

Diagnosis:
- Neuropathy of the tibial nerve and peroneal nerve on the right side
- vague soft tissue inflammation around the hollow of the knee on the right side.

Treatment:
- operative exploration of the right tibial and fibular nerves and of the sciatic nerve.

Ms M. was transferred to the neurological department of the University Hospital where the operation would be carried out.
- No lesion was found intraoperatively, no inflammatory or tumorous formation.
- Neurological symptoms unchanged.

Treatment:
- Fitting and receiving a peroneal splint (due to weakness of dorsal flexor)
- Physiotherapy
- Painkillers and antidepressants

The pains persisted and there was no improvement in mobility … When Ms M. was with the shoe technician, Mr R., who was preparing special inlays for her children, asked why Ms M. was wearing the peroneal splint. After she explained her case history, the assiduous shoe technician examined Ms M.'s right foot and recommended that she remove the splint immediately, or the anterior tibialis would degenerate further. The technician also recommended that she should go to an orthopaedic doctor to obtain a prescription for orthopaedic shoes because of the splay-foot, and the possibility of arthrosis. Ms M. took delivery of the orthopaedic shoes in December 2008 and from that point on, walking was easier. But the pains persisted, and were unbearable at times.

The doctor prescribed Matrifen painkilling patches to keep the pain in check. The active agent is Fentanyl which has very unpleasant side effects, among them the danger of addiction. This medication is usually only used to combat extreme pains, mainly tumour pains that cannot be alleviated by any other medication. By pure coincidence Ms M. met a woman who had been cured of severe arthrosis pains. She told Ms M. to contact Mr G., which she did. He told her about DMSO (Dimethyl sulfoxide) and MMS, how they work and how to take them, and gave her the medicines. Mr G. was uninterested in making money and did not want to profit from it. He had once been very ill himself and wanted to help others as did Jim Humble, whose book he strongly recommended she read.

There was a significant improvement after using DMSO and MMS. The pains disappeared after only a few applications of DMSO on the painful areas. A further improvement came about after she took MMS. Ms M. could now resume her household tasks without difficulty. She does not need any painkillers, antidepressants, or Matrifen painkilling patches …
Many thanks to Mr G. and to Jim Humble; everybody should read his book.

02/08/2010: Helga Scheibe from Lemgo. Recovery from various ailments.

I took MMS for three months, ultimately taking ten drops a day (after the first month I took 13 drops a day for about two weeks). I started on 26 April and stopped taking it temporarily on 24 July 2010. Clear improvements: • I could sleep better. • My gums became firmer. • My head became clearer. • Vague pains around the abdomen (lower stomach and kidney area) decreased. • A cough that had persisted for one year receded.	*Sleep disorders* *Gum problems* *Stomach aches* *Cough*
When visiting me, my eleven-year-old grandson was stung by bees twice on the flat of his foot. Instant recovery: I dabbed the spot with 30 drops in 100ml of water. I stopped taking the medicine because I 'dreaded' it. I found the smell intolerable and the acidity nauseating. I never mixed it with juices, I didn't want to 'cheat' my senses. I had the feeling that the acidity crystallized in the muscle tissue. I had pains in my right shoulder; that could also, however, have been caused by working in the garden. The pains are gone but the work continues. I now feel relatively well (compared with before taking it).	*Bee sting*

4 • Remarkable therapeutic successes

28/08/2010: Barbara Berends, 53 years old, from Emden

Anal itching — I had had an incredible itch in the anal region for a few weeks, most notably at night, in a warm bed, and when it started I wouldn't be able to control myself and would scratch it until it bled. I made a test mixture from MMS drops and drank it. It was a mixture of three drops per bottle. The itch disappeared within 24 hours and has never returned. After a week I had my own stock of MMS and I took this in slowly-increasing doses for ten days – to clean out my body, so to speak. I am taking a break from it now because I have some problems with breathing and because I am not sleeping particularly well. I'll take it again after a break.

On 13/01/2011 she added:

Warts Virus — A thick wart had developed on my chest. I mixed one drop from each of the bottles and let it activate. Then I soaked up the yellow liquid with a cotton wool pad and dabbed the wart with it. I did this every morning after showering, and ten days later all that remained of the wart was a tiny little mark.

My son-in-law had caught a cold. The doctor said it was a virus. He took MMS three times a day, four drops each time, and after three days he could smell, taste and was healthy again.

06/09/2010: Monika K., Bavaria

Urinary tract infection
Candida
Toxoplasmosis
Borrelia

I had a number of pathogens during a phase when my immune system was weak. Candida, toxoplasmosis, the remnants of borrelia, and a virus that affected the urethra. After taking MMS in an initial self-experiment for three weeks my doctor, to her great surprise, could no longer find any indication of them. However it took another few weeks before I felt well.

12/09/2010: Ulla M., Munich

Thyroid nodule — On two weekends when I had nothing planned, I tried taking a mixture of 16 drops (divided into 2 x 8 drops due to the taste) in the morning on an empty stomach for two days running. This had a very positive effect, especially on the tension in my muscles, but it was extremely uncomfortable and I had to deal with bad diarrhoea and flatulence for days after this high-dose intake. I have now gone back to a daily dose of eight drops in the morning and eight in the evening, which helps noticeably but is somewhat slower. The advantage is that it causes significantly fewer stomach problems and is therefore more bearable.

Muscle tension

This week, the roof of my mouth was badly inflamed as were the interspaces of the gums. Using dental floss was extremely painful so I made a mixture using six activated drops, added some water and took three mouthfuls, one after the other, which I swilled around my mouth for about a minute each. The inflammation disappeared after two days; only one spot on the back molar still hurts a little. I noticed a pleasant side effect: the dark plaque stains on the edges have shrunk. I have decided to continue with these mouthwashes after brushing in the morning and evening. We'll see how that comes along.

Gum infections

Dental plaque

My thyroid nodule continues to shrink. I have a check-up appointment with the internist next week. I am excited to see what comes of it. I'll be happy to let you know.

The only unpleasantness is the condition of my hands. Unfortunately, I can't detect any further improvements to the knots. But even if it remains as it is now I can manage without an operation, which is a great help.

06/10/2010: John G. from Great Britain prayed for his girlfriend who had cancer and heard about MMS.

My girlfriend had lymphatic cancer. She was close to death and the only things keeping her alive were her willpower and positive attitude. She got through the chemotherapy but was hurting all over. Her condition was so bad that the doctors told her after the eighth chemotherapy cycle that she should have a scan to see how it looked, and then start radiotherapy. I told her about MMS and she started with 5 drops x 5 times a day after her last chemotherapy. When she had a scan a month later, the doctors who did the tests were shocked. They couldn't find anything. There wasn't anything left to be radiated. There was nothing left of the cancer.

Lymphatic cancer

She felt better each day and the pains in her body receded. No one at the hospital could believe it, neither could her family. She was so happy! After all, she had already prepared herself mentally; she had known that it could all come to a terrible end. I want to thank you on her behalf and tell you how indebted I am to you because I love this woman so much that I prayed to God that he would provide a miracle and make her well again. I will certainly be telling others about MMS. I was told by a relative who is a doctor that the content of MMS is harmless compared to other medications we use that have several side effects.

01/10/2010: Sent by Ann Schneider-Cullen; Leon E. from Great Britain feels like a new man.

General detoxification

I bought MMS 1 and started taking the drops morning and evening. I wanted to really detoxify my body so I increased the dose quickly. That was not a good decision because too many poisons got moving too quickly. I felt sick quite often and I had lots of diarrhoea. When I reached six to seven drops I had bad diarrhoea for three days and felt pretty weak. I now know that I was pushing myself too hard and that that was not necessary. I recently bought MMS tablets and that was much better: no diarrhoea and no nausea.

Now that it is all over I feel really very good, physically as well as mentally and spiritually. I definitely feel purified, my energy levels are higher, and my sensory perception is better. I am more aware of all the bad stuff I am putting into my body, such as when I drink tap water which smells like chlorine. I never noticed that before. Ann explained that this is one of the results of detoxifying my body. My body is now more sensitive. I would advise everyone on this planet to take MMS. The only way I can describe the feeling I had after recovering is that it is like being born again. I feel like a new man!

10/10/2010: Ursula Tasche, Heiden

Chronic stomach aches

I had constant stomach aches for over ten years, sometimes severe, sometimes less so – it hardly responded to treatments at all. After taking MMS for a few weeks they disappeared. I started with three drops and increased to 15 drops within 14 days.

Experience reports

16/10/2010: Ms E. S., Lippe

I suffered from bronchitis for years, in summer as well as in winter. MMS was effective for me in the following ways:
took it mornings and evenings for 3 weeks. Started with one drop, increased during that period to eight drops, but only took eight drops once, then only took six drops for many days because I had an increasing aversion to it. Daily soft stool, even diarrhoea and nausea. Result: bronchial cough much reduced as the bronchia cleared. Now, one year later, no sign of regression. Every two or three months I take three drops morning and evening for three to five days as a preventative measure.
I rinse my mouth and gargle with one or two drops every morning to help with oral hygiene.
I treat various cuts, wounds and abrasions with a drop diluted in a quarter of a glass of water, with excellent results. I treat itchy eyelids in the same way. A friend of mine had stomach pains after drinking milk. These completely disappeared after she took MMS for 14 days, as did a number of other minor complaints. I can heartily recommend MMS and will continue to experiment with it.

Chronic bronchitis

Cuts

Wounds

Stomach pains

20/10/2010: Heidrun Eibl, Kempten

I have been taking MMS for a few days now and I am very impressed by the effects.
I have suffered from diabetes for 43 years (since my first pregnancy) and have had to inject insulin for the last 15 years (3–4 times daily): a fast-acting insulin, and a slow-acting insulin overnight. I have suffered severe leg pains for the last few weeks – either one of the delayed effects of my diabetes, or referred pain from my back (I have had back pain and arthrosis in a number of joints for many years). Yesterday however I was able to go to sleep without pains in my legs for the first time in weeks – a wonderful feeling. Added to that, as a precaution I have only been injecting 13 units of slow-acting insulin instead of the usual 15, and I have good levels in the mornings despite that. This morning I also took one unit less of fast-acting insulin and already 1½ hours before lunch my levels were almost hypoglycaemic. I think that is great. I woke up completely fresh this morning and had slightly less back pain than usual. I also feel better in other ways. However, I have to admit that I took two drops from the very beginning. MMS

Diabetes

Leg and back pains

Arthrosis

Gum infections

has had another positive effect. I have often had gum infections and on my dentist's recommendation I tried 'oil swishing' for a few weeks: swilling your mouth with a tablespoon of sunflower oil for about 15 minutes, 1–3 times a day, before spitting it out. This is supposed to decrease the amount of bacteria in the oral cavity. It actually worked to a certain extent, but since I have been taking MMS the inflammation has disappeared.

22/10/2010: E. S., Schleswig-Holstein

Metastatic rectal carcinoma

In March my husband Wilfried was diagnosed with hepatic metastatic rectal carcinoma. An operation followed and my husband was given an ileostomy. My husband was prescribed chemo due to the metastases in his liver. Weakened by the operation, my husband's condition was made even more precarious by the chemotherapy. He made the decision: no more chemotherapy. At the same time we heard about MMS and for us there was no mistake about it: that *is* an alternative. He started on 19/07/2010 with 2 drops x 3 times daily and increased the dose to 7 drops x 4 times daily by 02/08. He then increased it by two drops each day but started having diarrhoea. He is now staying at 28 drops and since September has been following the new protocol, spreading the dose over the day in a litre of water.

Today, after taking MMS for 4 months, my husband is in a stable condition. The last CT on 22/09/2010 shows that the tumour cells in the liver have stopped growing. A blood test on 30/09/2010 shows improved blood counts with a reduction in the levels of the tumour markers from 770 to 330. My husband is increasingly gaining in strength and is maintaining his weight.

21/11/2010: H. R., Switzerland

Flu

Colds

Lumbago

Toothache

I have been using MMS for more than a year, for myself and my family of three teenage children. The MMS solution has impressed some of my friends, who have also used it. I will list here some of the illnesses that we have successfully treated using MMS:

1. Early stages of common colds and flu-like infections. Taking three drops of activated MMS once or twice, and a good night's sleep, put a complete stop to the development of a cold.
2. Chronic, recurring lumbago for nine months was not really helped by

chiropractic treatment. Two doses of MMS brought on diarrhoea and the end of the back pains.
3. Since his last dental operation, my husband had been having toothache due to an infection in the nerve operated upon. Swilling his mouth with MMS and taking it internally for two days permanently freed him from the pain, which would have otherwise necessitated taking prescription painkillers for a week.
4. We treated our dog for cancer prevention. A tumour was removed four months ago. There is quite a high chance that metastases will develop in the liver or the spleen. We give him MMS in drinking-water as a precaution and hope for the best.

28/11/2010: Franz and Marianne Salinger, Paderborn

I first heard of MMS in May this year. After briefly reading up on it I soon forgot all about it. About six months later I came across some information about MMS again. This time I read about it in more detail and then bought the MMS drops, as well as Jim Humble's book. My husband began to read it carefully. We began to take the drops immediately (starting with one drop and then increasing) twice a day, but taking one extra drop in the evenings. The drops agreed with us and we felt well. My husband increased his dose to 15 drops three times a day, doing so for eight days. He had some diarrhoea on this dose, but it was tolerable. We continued to take MMS because we always felt cleansed and amazing. We now take 15 drops in the evenings and are stunned by the detoxification that happens overnight. My husband was examined by his GP before starting on the MMS and found that he had an elevated erythrocyte sedimentation rate. He also had numbness in his hands. Diagnosis: Carpal tunnel syndrome.

After taking the drops for three weeks he had more blood tests. The ESR was now back to normal and all other levels were fine. The GP could not explain why the levels had improved and suspected a laboratory error. The numbness in the hands has also lessened, with a warmth reaching the joints of the hands during the first days of taking MMS.

My husband has often been troubled with colds and inflammation of the sinuses and used to take Meditonsin. These symptoms completely disappeared after taking MMS drops for just a short time. The snoring has stopped. My husband's slightly but constantly raised blood pressure is now down to normal.

Elevated ESR

Numbness (Carpal tunnel syndrome)

Inflammation of the sinuses

Snoring

High blood pressure

4 • Remarkable therapeutic successes

12/01/2011: Susanne Schüttler

Chronic tonsillitis

Dry cough

Colds

Pollen allergy

Atopic dermatitis

Food intolerance

Excess weight

When I first heard of MMS eighteen months ago I had no idea how much it would change my life and that of my family. Back then it was the last modicum of hope I hung on to that I would be able to avoid a tonsillectomy. Some of your readers might regard it as a routine operation that is hardly worth worrying about, but I did not want to lose my body's 'health police' in this way. Anyone who has had chronic tonsillitis will know how unpleasant it is to constantly feel that you have something in your throat, to wake up every night with a dry cough, and to struggle with a cold almost every month. When I saw an open wound in my throat just above the inflamed tonsil, it was time to take action. Antibiotics had long stopped working and although homeopathic remedies brought some relief they did not bring about the breakthrough I was looking for. I ordered a generator to produce colloidal silver water and I saw Jim Humble's book *Breakthrough* for the first time in the advertising leaflet that was included. After reading the book, I simply had to try out the product; after all, things could hardly become worse.

And so in July 2009 I began to take MMS. The new protocols did not exist back then so I just started with one drop in the evening and increased the dose slowly. I took the MMS, activated it as instructed, morning and evening, and I experienced the unpleasant side of MMS for the first time when taking 5 drops. I also noticed how urgently my body needed this detoxification. The first thing I noticed was that I did not catch colds as often – things were looking up. Last summer I was able to pass by a meadow without sneezing once. It was only then that I really noticed that my pollen allergy, which I had had for 25 years, had disappeared. In the meantime I've changed to the protocol whereby you take a small dose of MMS eight times in eight hours. And I bought a kinesiology rod, which was more than worth the money. I can now find the correct dose very precisely by asking simple questions. It has also revealed that it is not only my tonsils that are infested with bacteria but my liver, my heart, and my lungs too.

Since shortly before Christmas I have been able to eat everything (I had food intolerances) and am free of allergies once more. The bacterial load in the lungs and heart has already disappeared, and that of the liver and tonsil is constantly decreasing. My body will be completely detoxified in about four months. And, as an aside, my weight is returning to what it should be for someone of my height – all without going on a 'magic diet'. You really notice when overburdened organs, such as the liver, are able to perform their tasks again.

After doing a kinesiology test I gave my daughter (7 years old) MMS and she was fully detoxified within a few days; it got rid of all her allergies, she doesn't have atopic dermatitis any longer, and she's as fit as a fiddle.

Even my son (2½ years old) is now given MMS to bring out the poisons from all the vaccinations.

I have also 'prescribed' three drops three times daily for my husband so that he can be rid of his persistent helicobacter infection. I can only recommend not giving up immediately if people see no results during the first few weeks. Our bodies are a synthesis, after all. So many little things are affected without us being aware of them – before we really feel an illness. But what is a year or two, compared to a lifetime of being dependent on doctors, pharmacies, and chemical medications that fail to make people truly healthy?

After all, MMS (in appropriate doses) only harms the bad things in your body. My intestinal flora is in good shape, which is not the case after a few days on antibiotics.

12/01/2011: Elke S., 46 years old, Bad Oeynhausen

I have been taking MMS drops for about 6 weeks – I am astounded by how quickly it takes effect. I have been suffering from bronchial asthma for years and can't really leave the house without my inhaler. I noticed significant improvements soon after starting to take it. The number of inhalations I need is already down by half. My skin's appearance, although I suffer from atopic dermatitis, is beginning to improve noticeably – patches that used to be dry and itchy have disappeared or have been reduced significantly.

Asthma

Atopic dermatitis

14/12/2010: Claudia Siedl

I am 44 years old and have had lichen sclerosus for about three years. It is an autoimmune skin disease that is, according to orthodox medicine, incurable. The skin tissue destroys itself, and becomes like porcelain: thin, whitish, and itchy …

It can appear over the whole body or on the genitals – I had white, itchy skin patches on my clitoris … I could keep it well under control using almond oil mixed with tea tree oil and lavender oil … I had to apply the oil to the affected area about four times a day to keep the itching at bay; at night, it was more severe due to the warmth under the duvet, sometimes I woke up at night …

Lichen sclerosus

Itching

I have been using MMS for about five weeks, and have increased the dose to eight drops as instructed in the book … At the same time I have been applying a weak spray solution, which has already given some relief … I once applied pure MMS onto my vagina four times; it burned a lot but was somehow more pleasant than the itching … it got pretty raw after that … and since then I have just been bathing twice a week in 30 drops of MMS with double the amount of activator (increased from 10 to 20, then to 30) – I have the feeling that MMS is absorbed into the body through the skin … I am always tired afterwards … detoxified probably … the itching has completely disappeared since then.

I can eat everything again: sugary, spicy, and salty food made the itching worse before. My digestion has also benefited … I did, however, suffer from dry, itchy patches around the corners of the eyes – in Chinese medicine the eyes are linked to the liver – and I interpreted that and the enlarged lacrimal sacs (kidneys) to be part of the detox process during the intensive, high-dose phase … It is gone, now that I am only bathing in it twice a week …

By the way, I stopped taking it immediately after eight drops because it was disgusting …

I tried to fill capsules with it and swallow them, but that also felt 'sharp' in my stomach …

Being able to eat everything and to live without itching has made an enormous difference to the quality of my life.

I don't know whether or not I am healed; the only test available is a punch biopsy, which I would never do. But it is no longer detectable in the blood … I am free of itching again and I only continue to bathe in it for general detoxification … the whitish areas are still there, maybe a bit weaker – time will tell … I don't use shampoo any more and my hair and scalp have changed since MMS … I go longer without washing my hair – no itchy scalp.

28/11/2010: sent under the initials 'E. M.'

Leg ulcers (Ulcus cruris)

Heart failure

High blood pressure

Ten years ago, my husband (70 years old) underwent the first operation to strip varicose veins with the result that he probably contracted MRSA; the leg would not heal, and when it did it would open up again after six months at the most. Five years ago he had the first defibrillator implanted because of heart failure: reputedly a heart function of only 20%. He went to the clinic in the spring of this year. He was to have a skin transplant on two open wounds on his leg. The result, five weeks later: he was laid up in bed with six open wounds on his leg; the feet swelled up badly after getting up for the first time and turned dark blue. Doctors' opinion: 'We can't do anything more to help.' He was given a wheelchair and that was that. Since I (70 years old) have been giving doctors' surgeries a wide berth for a number of years, I persuaded my husband to hand all 'antihypertensive' medication back to the doctor. I did some research online and came across the MMS and Strophanthin websites. We've been using it ever since, even giving our dog MMS, Strophanthin and hawthorn tea. My husband and the dog are now in great shape, and I was well in any case. The ulcus cruris is completely gone. No sign of high blood pressure. We go for walks of at least an hour every day, and drive around Europe in the camper van.

12/02/2011: sent by Elisabeth W.

Ten years ago I had severe problems with my lumbar vertebrae (sliding vertebrae) and they told me that there was no question of operating on it since it was inoperable. I would be in a wheelchair by the time I was 50 or 60 in any case, they said.

Prognosis: wheelchair

I am now past 50 and this problem made itself very noticeable in October 2010. I had severe pains when getting up and starting to walk, and could only walk very slowly. Climbing up stairs was also very painful. A friend of mine told me about MMS in January 2011 – she had also only just heard of it. She had been suffering with her jaw and teeth since she was 14 years old (constant suppuration). We both decided to try taking six drops (x2) of MMS hourly. Neither of us was very sure of this, but we told ourselves if it is supposed to help, then we would have to see it through for a few days. I felt a slight improvement on the next day and climbing the stairs was no problem. In my friend's case, the puss was really flowing and the pains were less intense.
I then bought Leo Koehof's book *MMS – Krankheiten einfach heilen* [MMS – Curing Disease with Ease]. I was and am sold on it and I decided to do the three-week regimen (3 drops of MMS and 3 drops of 50% citric acid every hour for 8 hours each day). Today is the eleventh day and I am completely stoked. Before I drink the solution I dip my fingers (after cleaning them) into the glass and massage the nails – they are becoming firmer.
I no longer bite my nails, which I have been doing since childhood.
So much has happened since I've had MMS at home and it would take too

much of your precious time if I were to write about everything here. So I thank you from the bottom of my heart and I would welcome the advance of Jim Humble's MMS to the four corners of the globe.

Just one last thing: my friend used to smoke. She's given up since taking MMS because she no longer likes the taste – she's delighted. THANKS, JIM HUMBLE! Thanks for your work!

Addendum on 14/02/2011

Just another short note on MMS: it's fantastic – every day I notice how the pains become fewer and fewer.

18/11/2010 Monika S., Lippe

Wart I started taking MMS this spring as a preventative measure. I began by taking one drop, increasing to 10 drops, and then reducing the dose by one drop a day down to one drop. Then I took a break of about two weeks before taking six drops a day for two weeks. During this time I dabbed a wart with MMS twice and forgot all about it. Now, three months later, I'm surprised to notice that the wart I had had on my pubic area has disappeared.

16/02/2011: Antonia Socher, 85 years old

Tuberculosis

Asthma

I contracted tuberculosis of the lung 60 years ago and my left lung has been deteriorating gradually over that time and I've been spitting out some nasty stuff. The doctors operated on it, taking out seven ribs and implanting a wax plate. I was then given many penicillin injections. In the meantime, my left lung decayed completely and is no longer there. A few years ago I was diagnosed with asthma on top of it all.

I heard about MMS at about the time the asthma became unbearable. I took it for eight days. I increased the dose slowly from 2 to 15 drops. I had bad diarrhoea during this time, and mucus ran from my nose. My body was cleansing itself thoroughly. After ten days, just to be on the safe side, I went to the doctor for an examination. He listened with his stethoscope first on the chest, then on the back, and then on the chest again, shaking his head. I asked him anxiously what was wrong and he said: 'What have you done? Your lungs haven't been in such good condition for years. Whatever it is you have been doing, keep doing it.'

Case Reports from Doctors' Surgeries

October 2010: Sabine G., 47 years old, Bavaria

Before taking MMS, bowel movements only every 4–5 days approx. (chronic constipation). Taking Schüssler salts etc. did not help. Since taking 4 to 6 drops twice a day, the patient has had regular daily bowel movements without additional aids. The appearance of the skin has improved too.	*Chronic constipation* *Poor skin condition*

October 2010: Martin S., 49 years old, Bavaria

Mr S. suffered serious injuries to his right knee, and had an exposed bone, in a car accident eight years ago. Since then he has been suffering from chronic, movement-specific knee pain. After taking 6 drops of MMS twice daily for about two months there was no longer any pain. The pains in the shoulders – especially when playing volleyball – have completely abated.	*Chronic knee pain*

October 2010: Fritz G., 73 years old, North Rhine-Westphalia

Two years ago he had a basal tumour excised from the bridge of his nose by a dermatologist. According to the postoperative histology, the excision was incomplete. The relapse appeared to be clinical, meaning that another operation would be necessary. Due to the critical location of the tumour he was prepared to try treating the tumour with MMS. He took three drops diluted with water in a 1:1 ratio, soaked some cotton wool in it, and placed it on the affected area for 15 minutes, washing the nose thoroughly with water afterwards. After seven days, the affected area became raw and the skin peeled off. After 14 days the pigmented tumour disappeared, and the appearance of the preoperative scarring is improved.	*Basal cell carcinoma*

4 • Remarkable therapeutic successes

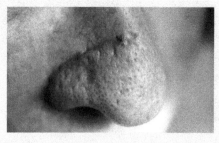

F. G.,
Basal cell carcinoma on the nose

F. G., sixteen days later

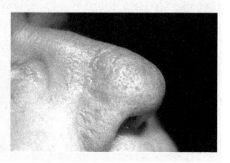

October 2010: Ms H. H., 70 years old, North Rhine-Westphalia

Aphtha   Ms H. is a severely disabled woman who presented with an aphthous ulcer of the oral mucosa. No subjective improvement could be detected after treating it locally with diluted MMS several times daily for three days. Because of this she took 2 drops of MMS with water orally 4 times a day. After three days (that is after taking a total of 24 drops), Ms H. was free of complaints and according to her nurse the aphthae healed.

October 2010: Lara S., 11 years old, North Rhine-Westphalia

Dog bites   The wounds were first treated using trauma surgery, followed by antibiotics as a prophylactic. The child's condition had worsened considerably by the fourteenth day. The injured cheek, including the upper lip and right eyelid, were very red and badly swollen. It was a classic case of extensive facial phlegmon.
The next day, the child was operated on by a maxillofacial surgeon. The surgical stitches were removed, puss rinsed from the wounds, and a swab from the wound bed sent for bacteriological testing. No microorganisms were found. The inflammation did not improve despite three days of intravenous antibiosis using Clindamycin. She had leukocytosis. The wound bed

was rinsed out and drained using disinfected iodoform gauze every day. Despite this, the child's condition did not improve. After using MMS (first day 1 drop; second day 2 drops; third day 4 and 6 drops; fourth day and onwards 2 x 6 drops) the inflammation was quickly reduced and was normal after 10 days.

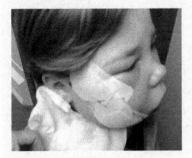

Lara, with a dog bite on her right cheek

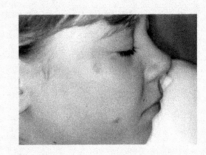

Lara, ten days later

October 2010: F. T., 5 years old, North Rhine-Westphalia

The child was bitten by a dog on the right cheek. In this case the bite wound was not treated surgically, or with any other medication, only with MMS applied locally (4 drops in 10ml applied to the wound every hour using cotton swabs) and internally (6 drops x 2 daily). The bite wounds healed within a week without becoming infected.

October 2010: Christoph S., 30 years old, Bavaria

Mr S. was overweight. After taking 6 drops of MMS x 2 daily, he lost 13kg within two months without changing his eating habits. He generally feels much better and has not had a cold since.

Excess weight

Colds

4 • Remarkable therapeutic successes

October 2010: Ms Brigitte S., 59 years old, North Rhine-Westphalia

Fibromyalgia

Chronic shoulder pains

Rosacea

Sleep disorders

Bleeding gums

Periodontitis

Seasickness

Ms S. took MMS (8 drops every evening) because of chronic shoulder pains that had lasted for months. The pains disappeared completely after three days. She also noticed that the rosacea on her cheeks was receding, and there were improvements in her sleep rhythms and general condition ('I feel bloody great!'). The bleeding in the gums of the upper jaw has abated (she lost the teeth in her lower jaw ten years ago because of periodontitis and regrets that she hadn't known about the drops back then). She stopped taking MMS because she felt so well. Three days later the fibromyalgia pain returned. Her sleep was naturally affected by that. So she started taking MMS again with the result that the pain disappeared immediately. A few weeks later she once again tried to stop taking MMS. The pain returned. She has now decided to take MMS regularly every evening for the time being because in this way she is free from complaints and knows that she has MMS to thank for that. She recently went on a cruise. When she felt seasickness coming on, she took five drops of MMS and felt well within 30 minutes.

She reports at the end of November that she no longer has any symptoms of fibromyalgia while taking MMS regularly.

October 2010: Mr J. D., 19 years old, North Rhine-Westphalia

Infection of the middle ear

Mr D. has been suffering from recurring infections of the middle ear since childhood; the infections consistently last for two to three weeks despite treatment with antibiotics. He had a bad infection of the middle ear while he was on holiday. His mother gave him eight drops of MMS in the evening and he felt a noticeable improvement within three hours. For the next two days he took a total of 24 drops daily, spread over the course of the day. The infection disappeared completely by the third day and he was able to enjoy his diving holiday without complaint.

The mother, Ms Brigitte D., 44 years old, North Rhine-Westphalia

Viral infection

Aphtha

Ms D. had a bad viral infection and despite intensive antibiotic treatment over three days, she could not get up from the sofa because her general condition was so weak. Her husband told her about MMS and so she took eight drops. Her condition improved within four hours. Three days later (taking 24 drops spread over the day each day) she was healthy again.

It took a week for her husband's illness to abate.

Ms D. often suffers from aphthae (usually lasting about two weeks; the aphthae were gone within two days of taking mouthwashes containing eight drops of MMS, and taking eight drops of MMS internally) and bladder infections, usually caught on foreign toilets while on holiday. After taking eight drops of MMS for two days she was well again and able to enjoy her holiday.

October 2010: Dr U. P. (female) from North Rhine-Westphalia is a hospital doctor

Ms P. suffered from a chronic infection affecting the vocal chords, and bronchitis, for three weeks. Various antibiotics brought no relief. She heard about MMS, did some research on the internet, and decided to take 24 drops spread over the day: 24 hours later the hoarse voice had returned to normal, and her general condition improved so much that she could hardly believe it. She thereupon recommended the MMS drops to other colleagues in her department. She also noticed that her immune system had become stronger.

Chronic antibiotic-resistant infection

October 2010: Jannik G., 11 years old, North Rhine-Westphalia

Jannik often suffered from protracted herpes infections that affected the whole mouth, throat and lip area. He stayed in bed for about two weeks, almost unable to do anything except sleep. He could not read a book and struggled to talk, eat and drink. He mainly drank sage tea and he treated his lips with sage compresses.

Protracted herpes infection

When he caught another herpes infection, he was treated using frequency therapy that included the whole face and throat area. Following that he tried a mouthwash with four drops of MMS. He swallowed a quantity of the solution that contained about two drops. According to his father, the swelling of the upper lip was much improved three hours later. The child was to take 12 drops a day diluted in a litre of water, spread over the course of the day. On the following day the child was able to leave his bed, and to take part in family life. Six drops of MMS were diluted in about 100ml of water and put in a spray bottle so that the affected genital area and hands could be disinfected. The child attended school on the fifth day and went to football training, although the lip was still not completely healed.

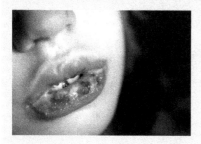

Jannik G., oral herpes

Jannik G., on day 7

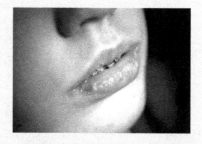

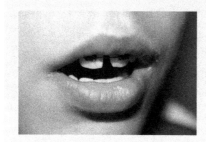

Jannik G., on day 14

October 2010: Siegfried L., 57 years old, North Rhine-Westphalia

Prostate cancer

Leg pains

Sleep disorders

Bisphos-phonates

Osteonecrosis

Mr L. is a 57-year-old patient who was given bisphosphonates intravenously over the course of many months to treat a bone metastasis of a prostate carcinoma that had been treated operatively as well as with chemotherapy. In Mr L.'s case, a necrosis of the lower jaw bone (left regions 36 to 38) developed. After unsuccessful dental treatment, he was transferred to a specialist jaw surgeon. He was reliant on walking sticks due to pelvic and femoral pains. Mr L. was told about MMS and took 30 drops a day, three weeks before the planned operation on his jaw. The necrotic lower jaw bone was removed and an anaplasty procedure sealed the remaining bone using autochthonous mucous membrane. No antibiotic follow-up treatment was given. The stitches were removed 14 days after the operation. The wound had healed without trouble or dehiscence. The pains around the pelvis and legs had also abated, leaving Mr L. able to walk without pain and without sticks.

To his great joy, the PSA levels fell slowly. He reports that he feels better now than he has done in a long time. His sleep is markedly better because he is not disturbed by pains in the extremities. He now takes 50 drops of MMS a day, spread over the course of the day, and tolerates this well; admittedly, he has been taking MMS with apple juice from the very beginning because he becomes nauseous when it is only mixed with water.

22/11/2010: Ms Rita H., 55 years old, Bad Oeynhausen

Ms H. has had trigeminal neuralgia of the second branch of the right infra-orbital nerve for six years in the form of regular 'attacks'. She usually had three or four of these attacks a day, which were excruciatingly painful. Then for eight months, starting in March 2009, the attacks occurred more frequently, coming on about 20 times a day like salvoes, leading to depression. Trigeminal neuralgia pains are among the severest pains known. Medicinal treatment (strong painkillers) and physiotherapeutic treatment had no significant effect. Reflexology massage was very painful. The pains were so severe that staff at the hospitals of Heidelberg and Minden suggested that she undergo an operation to have the nerve severed. Such an operation is fraught with risk.

The patient took twelve drops of MMS, spread over the course of the day, for two weeks, and took a bath with 15 drops of MMS once a week. She is now rid of her complaints and is overjoyed.

Trigeminal neuralgia

Extreme pains

Depression

When the publisher contacted her on 24/01/2011, she added:

Until now I still haven't had an 'attack'. I need to learn how to forget this constant fear that they will return.

For many weeks during the acute phase, I couldn't drink, eat, brush my teeth, put cream on my face, or blow my nose without having to reckon with the onset of an 'attack'.

I had forgotten how to laugh. I ignored the doorbell and the phone because facial expressions led to the attacks. I didn't leave the house for months because a slight breeze caused an explosive sensation in my face.

Activities with my family were kept to a minimum. I could only overcome the constant fear that these salvo-like blows would befall me in public by taking tablets to calm myself.

I am still careful in cold and windy weather.
I enjoy going out with my husband again, and playing with my grandson without fearing that he's going to grab my face.

More from Ms Rita H. in Bad Oeynhausen

My father has been dependent on nursing care for ten years.
He spends 22 hours a day in bed. He is fed by tube. He is actually a content old man, except for the constant nausea. Having had such a good experience with MMS, we have been giving him 3 drops of MMS twice a day through the feeding tube for the last seven weeks.
His nausea disappeared after four weeks and he could take a more active part in family life again.
He turned 80 last Monday and he celebrated his birthday with 55 guests.
What's more, my 3-year-old grandson spent the last year of kindergarten with constant coughs, colds and fevers. He caught every illness going around. He has been taking three drops every evening since November 2010 and hasn't even had a runny nose since.

August 2010: Ms C. B., North Rhine-Westphalia

Periodontitis

Loose teeth

Ms B. was complaining that the fourth molar on the upper left side was dangling like a cow's tail and was only hanging on by a thread. She couldn't eat any solids whatsoever because any chewing motion hurt badly. The gum was inflamed. When I told her about MMS she wanted to give it a try. She began immediately with a dose of 2 drops, twice daily. She also swilled her mouth three times a day with two drops of activated MMS in about 10ml of water.
The pain was noticeably better after the first mouthwash. By the second day Ms B. could chew foods almost without pain when doing so with care. In a few days she was chewing normally, the tooth was much firmer, and there was no more talk of extracting the tooth. Ms C. B. was pleasantly surprised since she had not held much hope that anything could be done to reverse severe periodontitis.

November 2010: Mexico

A woman from Mexico who works with autistic children has 55 children under her supervision who take MMS. Some of them have begun to talk, and others started doing things they had not done before within 70 days of taking MMS.
If necessary, contact her (in Spanish or English) via the website www.autismo2.com

Autism

11/02/2011: Hans M. from Glückstadt, frequent need to urinate at night

Dear Antje, I began taking MMS at the beginning of July 2010 because of my need to urinate at night. I increased the dose from one to eight drops twice daily. After about a month the need to urinate decreased. Since taking MMS, instead of going to the toilet three times a night, I only need to go to the toilet twice, maximum. And when I take a teaspoon of pumpkin seed oil in the evening (in combination with MMS) I only need to go to the toilet once.

Nocturia

17/02/2011: Diethelm Schmittat from Kaufbeuren

My wife and I experimented with MMS: we started with two drops, increased to seven drops by the seventh day – and that twice a day – and brought this first experiment to an end after 18 days. I was very surprised when my wife showed me the state of her legs. She has had varicose veins for over 30 years, one of which is in the hollow of the knee and is 8mm high. We were both so surprised and delighted that I wanted to write to Mr Peter to share our news, and that is how I came to write this letter to you today. MMS had one adverse effect: our bowel movements are not as regular as they were before we followed the regimen. But we have that under control now – by using sodium sulphate. If you have had other similar experiences I would be very grateful if you could let me know. (Author's note: until now I had not heard of constipation after taking MMS.)
I wish you all the best and that MMS finds a bigger market than it has so far. The raised veins on my wife's legs were all level after 18 days.

Varicose veins

10/12/11: Addendum by Diethelm Schmittat from Kaufbeuren

If you publish my letter, please bear in mind that it all depends on the constitution of the individual. I would at all events advise people to take three to four drops over the 18 to 28 days and observe carefully how MMS affects you.

I hope to have been of service with my empirical experience.

23/02/2011: Angelika Vanden Broucke Bergemann from Brussels

Tooth root inflammation with abscess

I have been treating my whole family with MMS for almost three years; myself, friends, animals and plants. Here are some of the successes I have had over the last few years.

I have treated tooth root inflammation with abscesses, both mine and my husband's. In each case the affected tooth was higher than the row of teeth and appeared to be no longer firmly anchored in the jaw. Normally this would be a case for the dentist, and root canal treatment. We treated it with MMS for two to three weeks and now the tooth is firmly rooted once more and the abscess has cleared.

Bleeding bladder infections

One of our dogs had been suffering from her recurring, bleeding bladder infections and treated with strong medications for years. Since she could not tolerate the chemicals any longer she became the first patient that I treated with MMS. I had read a lot about MMS but didn't know anyone personally that I could discuss it with, and so my knees were shaking when I put the first activated drops into the dog's mouth using the pipette. (Because my MMS comes from a first-class laboratory in which there is only the water purifier, I was confronted with the bright red warning: 'Danger to life when taken [undiluted]'.) Our dog was back to full health within two days, and without any side effects. After taking the tablets she would always stop eating and would become quite emaciated.

Oral herpes

I have seen some great successes with oral herpes. Both my husband and daughter suffer from it at times and I keep a small supply of medical ointments for it in the refrigerator.

Unfortunately they don't really do much to help and the growth of the blisters just takes its inflammatory course. It is usually more than a week before everything is healed.

But not so with MMS. Prepare a mixture of four drops plus 20 drops of activator (10% citric acid), topped up with two to three centimetres of water after three minutes: apply this solution repeatedly to the affected area using cotton buds and everything quickly returns to normal. Usually there is nothing visible after two days.

I always cover the glass with a saucer; that way the content remains active for longer.

MMS is excellent against dandruff and eczema. After three treatments it no longer 'snows' down onto the shoulders. Those special shampoos don't stand the slightest chance … *Dandruff*

My dear neighbour, a 90-year-old lady, had colitis and a bladder infection a week ago. She took MMS because she trusts me and is very open to alternative health methods. She is as fit as a fiddle today. (She did, however, have cramps and bad diarrhoea last night, but she feels well.) Her feet, which have been swollen for many years, have reduced in size after taking MMS, and even their reddish colour has almost disappeared. *Colitis*

My beautiful, massive Ficus benjamini (commonly known as the weeping fig tree) suddenly had lice (a sticky discharge on the leaves). I quickly prepared a solution of 12 drops, topped up with ¼ of a litre of water in a spray bottle, and sprayed the tree three times at intervals. As far as I can tell, the leaves are no longer sticky. *Lice*

07/03/2011: Dr Luise Stolz, 33098 Paderborn

I am a doctor specialising in general practice, homeopathy and psychotherapy, as is the author of this book. Each one of us has deep convictions or fundamental principles. One important guideline for me is that I will always try out anything I recommend to others. That is not only true for orthodox medications, which I prescribe sparingly, but also for almost everything in the areas of alternative and complementary medicine. For example, I recently ate a large amount of bitter almonds every day for almost a year. This 'food' is a topic of hot debate in the media and online: some praise it for being very effective against cancer, while others believe it to be extremely poisonous. I felt great before, during, and after this period. You can find reports of some of my experiences, including dosage recommendations, on the webpages of the Biologische Krebsabwehr Heidelberg (a centre for alternative cancer treatment). *Detoxification*

Now let's turn to MMS. I had already heard about the miracle drops from a number of different sources when one day I spoke to Dr Antje Oswald about it, and about the fact that she intended to write this book. By telling me of her experiences she gave me the courage to try it out on myself. I prepared my own mixture. During a normal day's work at my surgery I usually drink between 1.5 and 2 litres of water and since I didn't want to have to do the activating process each time I made a solution with ten drops, I put it in a dark bottle with water, and poured myself a drink with my normal drinking-water. That went well for about four weeks. One thing did strike me, however: after about a week or two I had vaginal discharge which disturbed me initially since I come from a 'cancer family'. But my gut instinct told me that this was simply part of a detoxification process. And so it was: after 10 days everything was back to normal.

Then came the holidays. My friend, who is also well acquainted with MMS – but clearly had different information from me – explained that I should drink the mixture diluted in water directly after preparation. Since I was on holiday and felt that I had become used to it, I made a mixture using eight drops twice a day. It was then that I experienced the power of these inconspicuous drops: terrible stomach aches and smelly, watery diarrhoea. Initially I didn't even think of MMS – but on the third day it became clear that there was a connection between taking MMS and my ailments. I cut out the drops for four days until my bowels had settled and then started with a dose of two drops twice a day, which I tolerated well. I then increased this dose slowly – relying on 'gut instinct' – and that was fine. My experience: it is possible that considerable 'cleansing symptoms' will occur, that is, increased excretion of mucus, urine and stools, which, from a naturopathic perspective, is highly desirable and necessary for the healing process.

And secondly: if you, like me, find that you have recklessly taken an 'overdose', just take a few days off, start again slowly, and everything will run smoothly to the benefit of your health. I am very happy with the effect that MMS has had on my body. Since I was very healthy beforehand I can't report the disappearance of any health problems. But I felt excellent afterwards.

May 2011: Ms Joneikies from Düsseldorf

Pancreatic cancer

Ms Joneikies is a nurse who has worked in oncology for many years. Her negative experiences with chemotherapy drove her to look for alternatives when she herself became ill with cancer, and she decided on MMS. The pancreatic cancer was diagnosed by CT scan in January 2009. She began taking MMS in May 2009. She started slowly with one drop, and increased to ten drops each evening and an additional six drops during the day.

After taking MMS for nine months, she underwent another CT scan. The pancreatic cancer could no longer be detected.

She had felt that she was better a month earlier and the pains had disappeared. She did not undergo any treatment other than MMS during this time. She is still well at the time of writing (December 2011).

20/06/2011: Carolyn Czichos and Reinhard Kalus from Bamberg

We take MMS regularly for various minor health conditions such as periodontitis, skin or bowel problems, and we can see how it works in our bodies.

Periodontitis

Skin and bowel problems

My first intuitive impression was that MMS not only works on the physical level, but also on a higher-vibration mental level, or on the level of the air element. In my perception this corresponds to the chakra system (in contrast to the meridians or the astral body) on a human light anatomy vibration scale. MMS appears especially to brighten and raise the vibration of the individual chakras and, with regular use, the whole chakra system.

Brightening the chakras

So since MMS possibly works from a mental vibration level, I have the impression that this medicine can also contribute to a positive, clear, bright mental lifting of the personal aura as well as the collective human energy field. My intuition tells me that MMS could be sprayed above the head or applied to the skin as a liquid. This kind of effect could purify and bring serenity to the mental part of the aura, so that your thoughts become lighter and purer, comparable to the effect of a long stay at the beach, for example, which can cleanse the auric field thoroughly. Cleansing the mental aspect of the auric field in this way could help make it easier to perceive beings of positive light such as angels. Developing this idea further, MMS sprays could be used against all kinds of air pollutants and impurities. External application could include purifying chemtrails and pesticides as well as clearing old thought-form accumulations – such as disharmonious vibrations in interior spaces, on your property, in the neighbourhood in which you live, as well as to energetically lift places of power.

04/07/2011: Nina Rohlmann from Münster

Our meditation group came across MMS in 2008. We all decided to undergo a short course of self-treatment using MMS and most of us had diarrhoea

Cervical cancer

or vomited. I was the only one who had mid-cycle bleeding, which surprised us all. Then, during a routine gynaecological examination, I was diagnosed with cervical cancer and was to have an operation on the womb. (Although it should be noted that it was unclear how much would have to be removed.) I was 28 at the time and did not have children. I talked to my doctor and asked for six weeks to carry out an MMS treatment. If after that there was no significant improvement in the tissue, I would undergo an operation … It was now clear to me that the bleeding was a sign that the MMS had been trying to expel pathogens.

My mother and I set aside a whole weekend and I took MMS every two hours for two days [at a high dose]. At nights I only took it if I woke up, otherwise I allowed my body to rest.

Then on the third day, I took it every three hours, every four hours, every five hours etc. [a high dose] and gradually lessened it in a similar manner. I took eleven drops of MMS in the morning and again in the evening for a few more days. (I also did Peter Jentschura's alkaline vaginal washes three times a day for seven days.)

I would like to add that high doses of MMS should always be taken when there is someone there to hand, because for a while I felt very unwell and had become very weak. That is why I did the treatment with my mother at my side. Six weeks later, my doctor was astonished at the improvement in the tissue – a short time later and everything was healthy again. I am now down as a healthy patient.

That was three years ago. I feel great, and I am so happy that I avoided being operated on. What's more, no organs were removed and I can start a family.

06/07/2011: Peter Schmidt from Goldbach

Painful arthrosis

For a certain time I took MMS following Jim Humble's recommendations. I simply could not believe the effect this MMS was having. After a few days I noticed, almost daily, how the pains caused by arthrosis in the knees and foot joints abated. That was in the summer of 2010 – about six weeks after I started taking it. I have been free from complaints ever since and can race up the stairs at the grand old age of 60. Of course, it also cleared up a number of other little ailments.

I still can't quite believe it today. For me, MMS is more valuable than a gold ingot. I would recommend it to everyone, even as a preventative measure for those who feel well.

Experience reports

Luca S., 17 years old from North Rhine-Westphalia

Glandular fever

On Tuesday, 19 July, my son had a very sore throat and a fever that rose to 41.3 degrees during the night. Despite leg compresses and antipyretic syrup, his temperature stayed at and above 40 degrees until Friday. He was very ill, he vomited several times, could hardly speak, and the mucus in his throat caused problems. He underwent a frequency treatment against viruses and bacteria before taking MMS for the first time. He began taking the MMS drops on Friday; by Sunday the fever had dropped to below 39 degrees and he had an appetite for ice cream, which was the one thing he was able to eat despite having a sore throat – before then he had only drank tea and water, sip by sip. The sore throat continued to improve over the course of that Sunday, and by the evening he could eat solid food (pasta). On Monday the fever was down to below 38 degrees and he was able once more to get up to eat. On Tuesday, 19/07/2011, the fever and the slightly elevated temperature were as good as gone. All that remained was a certain weakness and exhaustion. I gave him four drops in a glass, three times a day for four weeks. From Saturday onwards he also bathed in the drops every second day. After taking blood tests at the paediatrician's on Thursday, 21 July 2011, and on Tuesday, 26 July 2011, the diagnosis of glandular fever was confirmed (with 99% certainty). The paediatrician was very surprised at the speedy recovery. Thanks to MMS, Luca was back in good shape within a few days (end of July).

04/08/2011: Beatrix Krause from Gräfelfing

Salivary stones

I have been doing a kidney cleanse for about two weeks – I drink a kidney-cleansing tea as recommended by Andreas Moritz. I have been taking MMS for eight days and have been increasing the number of drops each day without any nausea. I am at 3 x 12 drops today and only have slight diarrhoea. Over the weekend the parotid gland (salivary gland) became swollen; I had stones there – they worked themselves out.
That really is a fantastic result.
I am excited to see what else happens and what else my body will release!

4 • Remarkable therapeutic successes

12/08/2011: Dr Wolfgang Storch from Hermsdorf / Bad Klosterlausnitz, www.malaria-hilfe.de

Observations: black maculae

Three brown spots were slowly forming, one on top of the other, on the skin on my back. I sprayed them with chlorine dioxide water at irregular intervals. Then I applied a compress for about 24 hours, and kept it damp with 0.3% chlorine dioxide water. That led to a serious skin irritation that almost amounted to a cauterization. That area of skin regenerated itself completely within a week. I then observed that two spots were steadily becoming paler while the middle spot (about 6mm in diameter) was becoming darker. This spot began to grow relatively quickly over a period of three weeks. That would normally have been a matter for a dermatologist, who would certainly have surgically removed the spot.

I continued to dab the spot with a 0.3% chlorine dioxide water solution. On 4 August 2011 I bathed in the 12% salt spring mineral pool of Bad Klosterlausnitz (for 20 minutes) and following that, for 20 minutes in a sodium bicarbonate bath.

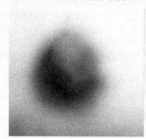

Figure 1

Then, I applied chlorine dioxide water compresses once more. On 7 August 2011, I noticed that the black spot had become detached from the skin. I tried to photograph this myself. In the evening I was able to remove the black skin parts, which caused a slight bleeding (Figure 1). I was able to stop the bleeding using chlorine dioxide. The skin then healed. Figure 2 was taken after more bathing in the Klosterlausnitz salt waters and in sodium bicarbonate baths. Now there is only a slight reddening on that area of the skin.

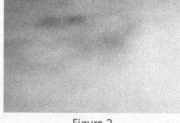

Figure 2

Figure 3 shows the formerly-attached skin. Despite the poor quality of the photographs, the images illustrate the successful self-treatment undertaken by using salt water and chlorine dioxide.

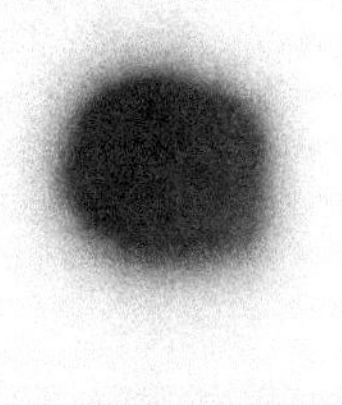

Figure 3

What I observed corresponds to other observations on the development of skin maculae, which I regard as the 'dumping grounds' of the body. The skin appears to have a self-protection mechanism and stores, in particular places, unpleasant metabolites that cannot be disposed of in any other way; these are distinguishable by their black or brown colour. When the ever-present need for self-purification of the skin is supported, then it is able to dispose of the accumulated toxins, a process I observed at first-hand.

Although other people had told me about such matters, I only 'half-heartedly' believed in the effects of chlorine dioxide water. I was probably meant to be persuaded of the astounding effects of chlorine dioxide water as a result of my own experiences.

Self-initiated skin cleansing happens very slowly. Some people lose patience and have the dark spots excised. The spots are then gone, but the necessary process of detoxification has certainly not been functioning. I still don't know whether or not that is now working well in my case. However, it is comforting to know that a black spot that was growing quickly, has disappeared from my skin with the aid of chlorine dioxide water.

28/09/2011: Anita Carapina from Voerde

One night my son, 13 years old, had an infection of the middle ear which did not respond to treatment. Heat, onion bags, pouring warm olive oil into the ear – all were done without success. *Infection of the middle ear*

Sometime around 3 a.m. I asked him whether we should try the new medication MMS. He agreed instantly. I activated a drop, diluted it in water, and dripped this into his ear. (I was a little anxious since I hadn't read anywhere that you could use MMS as an ear drop. But then I thought, if you can drink MMS, why not drip it into the ear?) One drop was enough. It didn't even take five minutes, I don't think. When I asked how it was, I got the answer: 'gone completely.'

After undergoing a 14-day MMS regimen the previous year (morning and evening in increasing doses), I went for 10 months without a migraine, and had headaches far less often than previously.

October 2011: Harm-Wulf Sluyterman from Denmark

My first-hand experiences of MMS:
- I often had aphthae in my mouth: MMS helped within half a day. *Aphthae*
- Severe pains in the big toe, probably gout, my father also had it, was gone within an hour. *Severe pains*

- Occasionally when brushing my teeth and to combat bad breath.
- For external injuries, for example inflammation caused by splinters.
- Two to three drops in a litre of water for my flowers; they grow fantastically well.
- A friend from Copenhagen had a fungal infection (candida) in his gut; his symptoms cleared within ten minutes of taking MMS and 1½ years later he still has not had a relapse.
- Two friends of my Copenhagen friend had genital herpes: cured after three days. That was a year ago and they are still free from complaints today.

Gout
Bad breath
Candida
Genital herpes

01/11/11: The Rasch Family from Bad Wörishofen

Nail and skin fungi
Skin impurities
Skin eruptions
Scars and wounds
Colds
Candida
Gum infections

We have been using MMS for about two years. During that time our whole family has been taking MMS for various illnesses (nail and skin fungi, skin impurities, skin eruptions, scars and wounds, colds, candida, gum infections) and as a result we have compiled a wide-ranging spectrum of success in the use of MMS.

Our home and travel pharmacy has effectively been reduced to a single medicine that can do everything.

But we don't just use MMS in emergencies, we also use it for general detoxification. We have been studying health intensively for a long time and are therefore aware of the importance of eliminating harmful substances from our bodies.

We are totally convinced of the effectiveness of MMS and a few weeks ago we even dared to give the smallest member of our family MMS. The elimination of environmental toxins, parasites and metabolic waste is not just an important topic for us humans, it is also just as important for our beloved pets. Jessy, our ten-year-old West Highland Terrier, has been taking activated MMS mixed in with her normal food every morning and evening for the last three weeks.

Jessy has never been given commercial pet food but has always been given lovingly-prepared food that is suitable for dogs. Over the passage of time our dog has become lethargic. We attributed this to her advancing age but we were put right.

Since Jessy has been taking MMS, fantastic things have been happening and we are delighted with these positive developments. All the supposed signs of aging have disappeared, and ticks that attach themselves to her are not able to suck blood until they get their fill: they drop off ahead of that. And we were able to stop the deworming medication with confidence since we have MMS to clear up parasites.

04/11/11: Josef Neuhold, Sankt Nikolai ob Draßling, Austria

I have some experience of MMS and I keep recommending it to others. It can be used to bring more or less any illness or complaint under control, when accompanied by a balanced, vitamin-rich diet that includes raw foods.

In spring 2008 I found out that I was lactose intolerant and I stopped consuming milk products. With this knowledge, and by avoiding this stressor, I noticed a number of positive improvements over the next few days: lowered pulse rate, relaxation, better sleep, more balance, clear skin ...

Lactose intolerance

I was significantly more relaxed as I went about my work because my stress levels had been appreciably reduced simply by excluding certain foods from my diet.

Initially it was absolutely no problem because the gains in quality of life easily compensated for the lost joy of nibbling. But sometime in the summer of 2008, I tried some chocolate (milk chocolate, of course). I reacted all the more acutely because my body was no longer used to this (daily) burden and I woke up on the following day with my head burning hot, and with painful swelling in the face and neck. It was really bad – and I was cured of my desire for chocolate for the time being.

I came across Jim Humble and MMS in September 2008 and I started experimenting on myself relatively soon thereafter. My logic was that stimulating the immune system by a multiplication of up to 100 – over 24 hours plus the anti-inflammatory effects – would neutralise the effect of dairy products (in my case, chocolate and ice cream especially). I started with six drops and increased the dose as instructed in the book to about twelve drops and maintained this dose over a few weeks to cleanse my body properly. I then reduced the dose to about six drops every other day (preventative) and I take MMS as soon as I get home if necessary, for example if I have eaten chocolate or ice cream.

The dose is between 12 and 15 drops, depending on how long I have gone without taking it. (High doses are not harmful but they can cause nausea and can have a laxative effect.) In contrast to before, or with low doses, I can stave off almost all discomfort. That is, despite eating chocolate, I sleep well all night, I wake up without any swelling, and the worst symptom I ever have is slightly unclear skin for a few days.

By now I have become used to it and MMS has increased the quality of my life enormously. With MMS I can now eat and enjoy whatever I like without worry.

Allergies to various shrubs and grasses

Incidentally, I have also been allergic to various shrubs and grasses for the last few years. In November / December 2008, I was keen to start on an allergy treatment in the form of drops; this would take about three months and I should be resistant by the time the pollen season started. I recently went to see the ENT doctor. Before ordering the special drops we did a new allergy test. The results were astounding: I no longer responded to shrubs and grasses that tested positive three years ago. Absolutely nothing! After checking the database I was asked whether or not I had taken any immune preparations in the meantime. The answer was NO – the cure could not be explained in that way.

I have had a number of corroborations from others since then because I am, naturally enough, completely convinced of the efficacy of these drops and am happy if I can help others to use them.

Painful inflammation

A good friend (45 years old, heavy smoker) fractured a bone in December 2008. He did not recover quite as had been hoped and they kept delaying the removal of the plaster. He then had a painful inflammation, and after two months he still couldn't put any weight on his foot. Having previously been very sceptical and refusing MMS, he tried it. It was really fascinating: the inflammation was gone after two days and he could then put weight on his foot.

Another case:

Severe joint pains (gout)

My aunt (past 60, retired nurse), has been suffering from severe joint pains (gout) for many years and takes a correspondingly high number of medications for the condition. Unfortunately they have yielded only minimal results, leaving her often unable to leave her flat. By now she has become open to alternative treatments and has tried the drops (December 2008). Since she found it difficult to drink the MMS due to the unpleasant chlorine smell, she was only able to increase the dose to eight drops. Despite that, after about two weeks she experienced a significant improvement and it has continued to this day. Her joints became freer and she can now move her fingers fairly well – the pain has reduced to a bearable level. A number of results – all positive – have occurred in the meantime, for example improvement of very critical blood levels in relation to the thyroid gland, and in another case in relation to the prostate gland etc. So simple and yet so effective.

07/11/11: Case reports from the alternative practice of Dr rer. nat. Hartmut Fischer, Lauterbach

Bee stings

Ludwig Sch. (6 years old) was attacked by a swarm of bees on 6 August 2011 and was stung about ten times. All the affected areas of the body swelled quickly and alarmingly, especially the face and neck because Ludwig has allergic tendencies. The family immediately asked for my advice because the boy was mentally very agitated. I recommended taking MMS hourly in accordance with the MMS 1000 protocol, a total of ten drops (in 1 litre of water). In addition, I recommended spraying the red areas of skin. The mother called a few hours later to report that the swelling had noticeably decreased and that her son, who had gladly drunk his hourly dose, had found relief.

Chronic constipation

Ms Miriam T. (29 years old) came to me in August 2011 to ask my advice regarding longstanding constipation. She had tried a number of laxatives without success and the painful constipation was leading to malnutrition with severe flaking of the skin on the hands, and to amenorrhea. I explained that it would certainly be wise first of all to detoxify her body after the sustained use of laxatives. In accordance with this recommendation, the patient drank an MMS 1000 solution (slow activation based on the Fischer method), three drops per hour, and after a few doses she developed severe nausea and diarrhoea. To her surprise, her digestive and bowel activity returned to normal. The patient admitted afterwards that at first she had not believed the medication would work at all. She also happily reported that she now enjoyed a healthy appetite and derived pleasure from eating. About three weeks later she went abroad for her summer holidays and on her return she complained that her bowels were sluggish when she boarded the plane. She wanted to take the solution again, and this time I recommended a lower dose to avoid the nausea. However, this did not yield the same results. Only when taking the original dose did the second treatment become successful and the chronic constipation disappeared. We are keen to see whether the other symptoms recede; this second treatment only took place last week.

Prostate cancer

Mr Karl Ludwig (64 years old) came to my surgery in June because, after a two-year battle against prostate cancer, he was regarded as being beyond treatment. The scintigram showed multiple metastases in the bones and lungs. A number of lymph nodes were palpably hardened / enlarged and the PSA levels were at 1562mg/mL initially (normal levels are 0–4 mg/mL). Mr Ludwig was in a sorry state and struggled to master the three steps to my front door. On my recommendation, he began to take the MMS 1000 solution (slow activation based on the Fischer method), which he quickly increased to eight drops per drink. However, this led to severe, roving pains. Although parallel measures were taken to support the liver, as well as nutritional changes / detoxification and appropriate physical movement in nature, the dose had to be reduced dramatically. Over the course of further treatment, he tolerated an MMS 1000 solution (slow activation based on the Fischer method) of two drops per drink very well. After about 2½ months, on 8 September 2011, his PSA levels came back at 193mg/mL. Mr Ludwig has been riding his bike again, has been making holiday plans, and buying furniture – in short, his perspective on life has changed. His breathing has improved considerably, and most lymph nodes in the head and neck area and in the groin are now normal. By now the PSA level has fallen to below 100mg/mL and the patient continues to take the specified MMS solution – doing so for five days, followed by a one- or two-day break, as suits his schedule.

21/11/2011: Heike and Manfred Romann from Wittlich

Malaria

I had been taking MMS on my own responsibility, and had had good results. So I recommended it to a friend, who is now my husband. He 'brought' malaria home from the war and has suffered numerous bouts over the last 50 years. He has written his story here:

'My name is Manfred Romann and I am 87 years old. I became a soldier at the age of 18, and after a short period of training I was sent to the Russian Front. In the spring of 1944 the Fronts began to retreat. At that time, I fell into the hands of the Russians and was put in captivity. We were loaded onto freight waggons, and we arrived at the camp after a journey of some days. Our camp was on the outskirts of Stalingrad. I worked there as a bricklayer and electrician. When there was no building work to be done they put us to work on anything they could find. And so one day I came to work for the "Waldkommando" whose task it was to fell trees. The trenches and the bomb craters were still there in this forest. As the snows melted and the river Volga broke its banks, the trenches and the craters filled with water. These were perfect breeding grounds for mosquitos. I was bitten countless times and became ill with malaria in the winter of 1948. I was just 24 years old. When I was no longer able to work I was released and sent home.

Over the next few years I had regular bouts of malaria, about two or three times a year. I had the shivers, fever, and fever-free periods. All this in turns. Over time, the bouts became less severe but since turning 70 they have gradually become more severe again. I simply cannot get rid of them.

One day a dear friend – who is now my wife – told me that there is a medicine for this illness. She called it MMS. I was sceptical at first but as I read Jim Humble's book I was won over. I began a cure regimen, starting with one drop a day and increasing to 15 drops. I stayed at 15 drops for eight days and then stopped taking it. That was about two years ago. Ever since I have been waiting for a relapse but nothing has happened. So taking MMS has been a great success. I am sure that it helps against other illnesses too. The malaria, certainly, has been cured.'

05/12/2011: Reinhard Kalus from Bamberg;
www.lichtwegegehenrkcc.de

I would like to point out once again that the tolerance threshold to MMS can be increased significantly by the addition of bicarbonate of soda. I received the following experience report from an acquaintance travelling in India:

'Many thanks for the tip regarding MMS. We had some very good experiences with MMS on our journey to India in 2009. We prepared our water with it and washed fruit with the water too. We survived the journey in good health. Some fellow travellers who were not so careful became ill. MMS got them back on their feet though.'

I wish you great success in disseminating this knowledge and in educating people regarding everything they put into their bodies.

05/12/2011: Paula from Bavaria

Impaired wound healing

Severe pains

On 9 December 2010 I slipped on ice and broke my ankle. I underwent an operation on it. The operation went well but after three or four days there was a problem with the wound – it simply wouldn't heal. The doctors explained that the tissue had died. I was treated with strong oral antibiotics (600mg Clindamycin active agent three times a day) for months without success. I had severe pains and could hardly walk. I came to know Mr G. through some coincidence via an acquaintance. He explained how to use MMS and DMSO. Following his instructions, I activated 30 drops of MMS and put them in the bath. There was an improvement after the first bath. I took an MMS bath three or four times a week, and dabbed the wound with 80% DMSO twice a day. Within 14 days the wound had completely healed. I would like to offer my heartfelt thanks for that and I recommend MMS and DMSO to everyone.

27/01/2012: Ali Erhan, 48 years old, Hannover

Food intolerances

Over-acidification

Fungal infection of the intestine

For over five years I have been suffering from lactose intolerance, severe gluten intolerance, very severe histamine intolerance with big, brown patches on my skin (mastocytosis = crystalline embedding of excess histamine in mast cells), constant and severe overacidification and many fungal infections in the intestine. After taking MMS drops hourly for two or three days, and increasing the dose each time, I can state that all my complaints and pains have abated by about 95%; I can eat bread and chocolate again.
www.HeilenmitMMS.de

February 2012: Ms Sophia P., over the phone

Child with Lyme disease

A two-year-old child suffering from Lyme disease was given three drops, three times a day (daily dose of eight to nine drops), in oat milk for ten days running. Following this the child was free from any symptoms.

4.1.2 Experience reports from animal owners

29/01/2010: Ms P.

My three-year-old dwarf rabbit had caught a cold. Constant sneezing and watery eyes. I gave the little one a drop in his drinking bowl and lo and behold, three days later it was better and the eyes were healthy again. He still sneezes from time to time, so he will still be given MMS for another week. It looks as if he likes it too, because his water bowl is empty every two days. I am thrilled! I also have a bad cold at the moment and have been taking MMS for a week (seven drops) and my cold is getting better, slowly but surely; most noticeably I can cough up again. I can only recommend MMS. Thanks!

Dwarf rabbit with a cold

09/06/2010: sent by Lothar Paulus

I have had two Rex mice with me at home for about six months and one of the two rascals has developed a tumour (which often happens with Rex mice). An acquaintance of mine thought I would have to put him down but I wasn't going to give up so easily on my Brainy (their names are Pinky and Brain) because I have grown very fond of him. Because I had had a few positive experiences with MMS myself, such as the curing of my constant reflux, I thought I would give it a try. My mouse's tumour had mushroomed and you could see and feel it clearly. In addition, blood came out of the little one's eye. I assume this was because the tumour was in the throat area. I have now been putting MMS in his drinking-water for two weeks and I could hardly believe it when, after a week, there was almost nothing to be seen any more, and he could see normally because the bleeding in his eyes had gone. He is now diligently taking food again, which he had hardly done at all before. You can hardly see anything now and I think I will have completely conquered this tumour in the next few days and that my Brainy will be with me for quite a while longer. I thank you from the bottom of my heart for this ground-breaking medicine. It has spared me and my mouse much suffering. The quality of my life has increased a great deal thanks to you. Eight years of reflux with extreme heartburn is now history. Where orthodox medicine failed, MMS gave me back my health.

Rex mouse with tumour

4 • Remarkable therapeutic successes

24/06/2010: sent by Britta E.

Tomcat with eye infection

We gave our tomcat MMS when our dog wouldn't stop chasing after him and yowling. He had an infection in one eye. I only gave him 1 drop of MMS + 1 drop of 50% citric acid. He was well the next day. Thanks to MMS I no longer go to the vet and I no longer have them vaccinated. I give them a drop a week as a preventative measure.

15/06/2010: sent by Lothar Paulus

Saved duck

Thank you MMS!
As I was driving along one Sunday I saw people gathered around a large, white duck at the side of the road; they were shaking its neck. Green mucus was being discharged. The duck was choking to death. I stopped and asked what was wrong with it. No one knew. I instantly thought of MMS and quickly drove home. Filled water into a bottle – cup – MMS – and off. When I arrived there I mixed the MMS. Topped it up with water – took the beak – poured some in slowly – the animal was slumped. I gave three drops – after ten minutes it lurched up, took off and waddled off towards the pond. I was so happy on that Sunday. I gave my telephone number; if there were any more problems I would come back to give it more MMS. I later inquired after the duck and it is doing splendidly. The people said I was sent by God. Thank Jim Humble, I answered. ;-) I have kept some MMS in my car ever since, just in case.

29/07/2010: Margita P., Lage

Tomcat with eye infection

Our tomcat Wob accidentally injured his eye on a willow stick while cavorting around – retinal tear. Medication: the homeopathic remedy ruta, antibiotic eye ointment and eye-healing salve. After a week, it was established that there was bacteria (chlamydia) present. Another week later and the tear had healed and only a dot was to be seen. The vet wanted to do bacteriological tests immediately because she was not satisfied with the effect the ointment had had, and the eye was not improving. I then thought of MMS so I stopped all the other medications. I gave the tomcat 1ml three times a day orally and dabbed at the closed eye carefully with MMS. After five days, the examination showed that everything was okay.

September 2010: Kerstin Depping, Lage

Dog with loose incisor tooth

My thirteen-year-old dog Lucky had an extremely loose incisor tooth that threatened to fall out. I gave her MMS for a week, starting with one drop of MMS and five drops of the activator, increasing to five drops. She tolerated it without problems and the tooth is now sitting tight in the row. What's more, she is now brighter, happier and generally fitter than before and we can take longer walks again thanks to MMS.

08/09/2010: Emma from England

Dog with tumour

I started to treat my nine-year-old dog with MMS on 10/08/2010 because it had a tumour in the abdomen. A few weeks previously they had told me, after laboratory tests, x-rays and scans, that my dog only had weeks, or a few months at the most, to live because of the tumour in the abdomen and the lung metastases. I gave him a two-dose pill every hour for eight hours (author's note: this is the MMS C30 homeopathic medicine in pill form, produced by the Ainsworth company, from a 28% technical grade sodium chlorite solution and 10% citric acid – probably produced synthetically – as an activator). I then continued with 4 x 3 doses and then with 4 x 4 every day. When I started, he wasn't eating normally; he could only tolerate cooked rice with liver and chicken. He could hardly walk, had lost a lot of weight, was lethargic, and had diarrhoea. Now, a month after starting with MMS, he is eating normally as before and has put on weight. He is very happy and is now going for walks of a normal length again. He has all the energy he had before his illness, and except for his swollen belly we would say that he is the same as he was before. The tumour was very hard, and it is certainly softer now. When we visited the vet recently he was very surprised and told me to carry on with whatever I was doing, which I intended to do anyway of course. I am very optimistic regarding his future and grateful that I found MMS because I am convinced that that is what caused this remarkable change in his condition.

October 2010: Richard from England

Dog with kidney failure

The vet diagnosed my dog with kidney failure and gave him just a few days to live. Two-thirds of his kidneys were gone. The lab tests showed that only one-third of his kidneys were still functioning. He really was very ill. We had been watching his decline over the previous six months. Two days before we took him to the vet he could neither walk nor eat. On the day I came back from the vet, I ordered MMS. It was a few days before it came and each day his condition worsened. As soon as we started to give him MMS his condition stabilised, then it became worse, before it stabilised again. That is how it was for a while. He was vomiting and had diarrhoea during this time, but we could see that his condition was gradually improving. It was difficult to increase the dose because he would usually become nauseous and couldn't eat much. But there was a real improvement after 14 days. He became livelier, started to eat his food and wanted to go for walks again, even if only for short stretches.

It is now seven weeks since we started treating him with MMS and he is sitting right next to me now and looks as if nothing has happened. He is walking his normal distances of three to five miles each morning and evening, and eating his regular portions at mealtimes. His coat is shiny and he looks two years younger than before. I give him a maintenance dose each morning and evening. It is all the harder to believe when you consider that he is thirteen years old.

14/02/2011: sent by Marion Schlenzka

Case 1: Mare with chronic laminitis

A dose of 120 drops a day was given to a mare afflicted with laminitis because the illness was acute and extremely painful. This dose was reached after increasing the dose from 30 drops to 120 over a few days.

The activated MMS was mixed with wheat bran and was quickly eaten without problem.

At no point did the mare's condition worsen, and she showed no signs of intolerance. On the contrary, her condition improved and improved and after a week she was able to walk in the meadow again.

Treatment was continued for four weeks at a dose of 120 drops a day, and then reduced to a maintenance dose of 50 drops a day. The MMS was administered in moistened wheat bran three times a day.

Today, the mare is walking and galloping happily in the paddock. She obviously feels better than before she became ill with laminitis. She is even allowed to graze, which was not possible previously because of her susceptibility to laminitis.

The owner had initially considered putting the horse down, especially after the last episode of laminitis because she had not come across any method of treatment. The horses suffer terribly from this painful illness. Administering MMS has saved her horse, and may possibly be a permanent cure.

The mare is now intermittently treated with MMS as a preventative measure, for example in spring and autumn, when there is greater susceptibility to laminitis; she is given 50 drops per day for four weeks. When a renewed episode of laminitis occurs, the high dose of 120 drops of activated MMS is administered.

14/02/2011: sent by Marion Schlenzka

Case 2: Horse with fist-sized hoof canker

This horse's hoof canker was as good as incurable and was threatening to lead to a detached hoof wall, which means putting a horse down. Inside, the hoof was soft and bloody, and the horse was hardly able to walk.

Thirty drops of activated MMS were diluted in about a litre of water every day, and nappies were immersed in it until they were fully saturated. These nappies were fastened onto the horse's hoof overnight and removed in the morning so that the MMS had time to slowly unleash its effect. This treatment stretched out over many weeks – at least six. Today, the canker has reduced to an abscess the size of a walnut and the hoof is in the process of regenerating itself. In the eyes of the blacksmiths and the vets it is nothing short of a miracle.

The treatment will continue until the canker is cured and the hoof has regenerated itself.

In neither case were there any signs that the animals felt unwell when taking MMS. It was also interesting to note that these animals were plagued far less by insects, gadflies and ticks in summer, in comparison to the animals that had not been given MMS.

12/7/2011: Peter Schneider from Spalt, Bavaria

Cherry-sized growth in the eye

Found while mowing the lawn – a three-week-old kitten – abandoned by its mother – dabbed with an MMS tincture every two hours – given to drink from a pipette – also mixed in with food – now, four weeks later, cat is healthy – everything okay – including the eye. Now the remainder of our team of cats also get some mixed in with their food. Dose: two drops activated in 40ml water.

October 2011: Mr A. G. from Bavaria

Bees with varroa mite

Parvovirus infection

I am still in the experimentation phase but I am very happy with the results. I add 36 drops of activated MMS to every 20kg of bee food. As a result, I have fewer mutations caused by bee viruses than would be expected for my 19 bee colonies, and there is no robbing between the bee colonies (which indicates that the colonies are in a good, robust condition), and I did not lose bees to the varroa destructor which has afflicted other beekeepers badly (cleansing flights, colony collapse, etc.). What gave me the idea of giving MMS to the bees was the fact that MMS had proved to be of great service to me and my family, and had quickly cured my seriously-ill dog of its parvovirus infection. I decided to try out MMS on my bees since oxalic acid, the treatment normally used to fight varroa mites, is also an oxidiser. Unlike Perizin and antibiotics it does not leave residues in the honey. I suspect that is also the case when MMS is mixed into the food and I will urge my colleagues to start their own experiments.

November 2011: Report by a Daniel-Peter-Verlag (Publishing House) customer

Healthier calves

I give each of my calves 20 drops of MMS in a litre of milk. Since I have been doing so my calves have become considerably healthier and not one of them has died. Isn't that wonderful? (Author's note: please note when giving MMS to calves that treatment should be discontinued immediately if they suffer from diarrhoea. See chapter 14 'MMS for Animals'.)

November 2011: A Daniel-Peter-Verlag (Publishing House) customer

Great results with doves

MMS helps with many illnesses in doves. In general, breeders see very good results when they regularly give the doves MMS in their drinking-water. The recommended dose is six drops of MMS in four litres of water. It takes about 14 days for the doves to get used to it, and to drink the water of

their own volition if they also have the choice of drinking rainwater.
Its effect is limited in cases of trichomoniasis.

Excellent, swift improvement was seen in cases of ornithosis, a parrot disease that causes lacrimation in the eyes, as a result of the following treatment: Administer 1 drop of MMS in 20ml water into the beak using a syringe (no needle) – it promptly helped.

Ornithosis, a parrot disease

Call for Contributions

We would like to thank everyone who has sent in reports regarding their experiences with MMS. We would also ask you, if you have taken MMS, to share your experience with us so that we can use those reports in future editions of this book or in a separate book – your experiences could help others.

The following points are important when describing your MMS experiences:

- Name the illness / diagnosis, or case history
- When did you start taking MMS?
- How many drops did you take per day?
- How many times a day?
- How many days did it take before your condition changed?
- In what way did your condition change?
- Do you have a doctor's report? Before / after?
- Please let us know if you would be happy for us to publish your story and whether we can include your full name. Doing so would allow you to credibly and convincingly highlight the efficacy of MMS in your experience.

Please contact:
DANIEL-PETER-VERLAG
Kirchröttenbach D 45
91220 Schnaittach
info@daniel-peter-verlag.de
www.daniel-peter-verlag.de

List of illnesses successfully treated using MMS

Sources: 1. Slide by Jim Humble; 2. Experience reports by users on the following websites www.jimhumblemms.de, www.mmsjimhumble.de, and www.jim-humble-mms.de; 3. Feedback from users

We do not promise a cure, neither do we claim that this list is complete. Jim Humble expressly emphasized this point in Mönchengladbach in 2010. In the meantime he has observed a number of other illnesses not listed here disappearing when MMS is used.

People with the illnesses listed below have, according to the reports, responded well to MMS. I cannot say whether it will help in your particular case, since each person's illness is such an individual matter.

Acne
Actinic keratosis
AIDS
Allergic bronchopulmonary aspergillosis
Allergies
Alzheimer's disease
Amyotrophic lateral sclerosis
Anaemia
Angina
Ankylosing spondylitis (Bechterew's disease)
Anthrax (splenic fever)
Aphthous ulcers
Apoplexy
Arterial blockages
Arthritis
Asthma
Atopic eczema
Atrial fibrillation
Avoiding transplants or subsequent problems
Back problems
Bacterial prostatitis
Bad breath

Bartonellosis
Basal cell carcinoma
Beta-thalassemia minor
Bipolar disorders
Bladder diseases
Blood diseases
Bone cancer
Bone metastasis
Bone, muscle, and connective tissue pain
Breast cancer
Bronchitis
Burns
Bursitis
Calluses
Cancer, various types
Candidiasis
Cardiac arrhythmias
Carpal tunnel syndrome
Cat allergies
Cataracts
Chickenpox
Chronic depression (dysthymia)
Chronic fatigue syndrome
Chronic kidney diseases

Chronic lymphatic leukaemia
Chronic obesity
Chronic pelvic pain syndrome (CPPS)
Circulation disorders
Cirrhosis
Colds
Complaints after transplants
Condyloma
Cramps
Crohn's disease
Cushing's syndrome
Cystic fibrosis
Dengue fever
Dental calculus
Depression
Diabetes types 1 and 2
Diarrhoea
Digestive difficulties
Diverticulitis
Earaches
Ear diseases
Eczemas
Emphysema
Erythema nodosum
Excess weight
Eye diseases and sight impairments
Fever
Fibromyalgia
Food poisoning
Fungal sinusitis
Fungal skin infections
Gastric ulcers
Glandular fever
Gout
Granulomatosis with polyangiitis
Gum diseases
Gum infections
Gums, bleeding
Haemorrhoids
Hair problems
Hay fever
Headaches
Heart attacks, idiopathic dilated cardiomyopathy
Heartburn
Heart diseases
Heart palpitations
Heavy metal poisoning
Helicobacter infection
Hemangioma
Hepatitis
Herpes labialis
Herpes zoster (shingles)
HIV
HPV viruses (warts)
Illnesses during pregnancy
Infections (of all kinds)
Inflammation of the breast
Influenza
Intestinal diseases
Irritable bladder
Irritable bowel syndrome
Jaw diseases
Kidney diseases
Kidney failure
Kidney infections
Kidney stones
Large intestine disorders
Leishmaniasis
Leprosy
Leucocytosis
Leukaemia
Liver diseases
Loss of hearing

4 • *Remarkable therapeutic successes*

- Lung infection
- Lung problems
- Lupus erythematosus
- Lyme disease
- Lymphoma
- Malaria
- Megaoesophagus
- Melanoma
- Meningitis
- Meteoropathy
- Migraines
- Morgellons syndrome
- Mosquito bites
- MRSA
- Multiple myeloma (plasma cell myeloma)
- Multiple sclerosis
- Muscle tension
- Myasthenia gravis
- Mycoplasma diseases
- Mycosis fungoides (TB-form with plate-like or ulcerous hardening of the skin, especially on the calves)
- Myoma
- Nail diseases
- Nausea
- Nervousness
- Nervous twitches and cramp in legs
- Nosebleeds
- Oedemas
- Oesophagus diseases
- Osteopenia
- Osteoporosis
- Osteosarcoma
- Ovarian cysts
- Oversensitivity to various substances
- Pancreatic cancer
- Paralysis
- Parasite infestation (also in pets)
- Parkinson's disease
- Parvovirus
- Pituitary gland tumours
- Poisoning
- Prostate diseases
- Psoriasis
- Q fever
- Restless legs
- Retinoblastoma
- Rubella
- Sarcoidosis
- Scarlet fever
- Scarring problems
- Sciatica
- Scoliosis
- Sebaceous cysts
- Sexually transmitted diseases (including gonorrhoea and syphilis)
- Shigellosis
- Sinusitis (sinus infection)
- Skin diseases
- Skin eruptions
- Skin impurities
- Sleeplessness
- Spinal stenosis
- Spots
- Stomach bugs
- Stomach cramps
- Stomach diseases
- Tapeworm infections
- TB

List of illnesses successfully treated using MMS

Tension headaches	Tumours, neuroendocrine
Tetanus	Typhus
Thinking, concentration, and memory disorders	Ulcerative colitis
	Ureter problems
Thrombocytopenia	Varicose veins
Thyroid diseases	Venous leg ulcers
Tinnitus	Vocal folds paralysis
Tiredness	Warts
Tonsillitis	Weakness, immune system
Trigeminal neuralgia	Weakness, physical
Tumours, cancerous and non-cancerous	Yeast infections
	Yellow fever

This list of illnesses that have been successfully treated with MMS might lead you to assume that it is a miracle substance that cures everything. I would disagree, and Jim Humble has never claimed that either. It is fairly certain that MMS cures malaria; at least I am not aware of any reports that indicate otherwise. It does what it can: it kills pathogens and detoxifies. Nothing more, nothing less. If that is enough to bring the patient back to health, they become healthy. If not, then not.

So if a cancer patient who has taken MMS is now free of cancer, it does not mean that that will be true in all other cases. If the cancer cells react sensitively to MMS, it could be the case, but that cannot be guaranteed. The only way for you to know if it works is for you to try it yourself – on your own responsibility. The same is also true for any other illness. As a doctor, I am not allowed to advise you to take a substance that is only officially approved for use as a water disinfectant, and not for internal use. But I would not advise you against it either. After all, many people have used it and have experienced an improvement in their health, or even a complete cure. And I would certainly not write a book about it if I were not happy with the effectiveness of MMS myself. However, a book cannot replace the trained insight of an expert. Therefore, if you suffer from a serious illness, it is certainly advisable to seek advice from a holistic doctor or alternative practitioner. You can still decide whether, when, and how you want to take MMS.

How to get hold of MMS

Jim Humble did not have MMS patented because his main priority was to make it available to everyone who needs it. He does not sell MMS himself.

There has been in existence a huge range of suppliers for some time now. See for yourself on the internet. If you enter 'MMS', 'CDS', 'Chlorine dioxide solution', or 'water sterilisers' into a search engine, you are certain to find a number of suppliers.

Health food shops You could possibly obtain a 0.29% chlorine dioxide solution (CDS) for water purification / sterilisation in the 'cleaning supplies' or 'personal hygiene' section of your health food shop.

In his book *Breakthrough* Jim Humble recommends using citric acid as an activator because it is more easily tolerated than vinegar, and because vinegar is contraindicated for those with candida infection. Users have discovered that utilizing tartaric acid or hydrochloric acid as an activator produces a pleasanter taste, and they are better tolerated. Jim Humble now only recommends the use of a 5% hydrochloric acid as an activator so that user results can be compared according to a standardised method. Depending on individual tolerance, I recommend using a 3–5% hydrochloric acid or a 50% tartaric acid as an activator. Citric acid, which is often produced artificially from the mould fungus Aspergillus niger, frequently leads to intolerance so I only recommend using it if you live in countries where hydrochloric acid or tartaric acid is hard to come by.

What you need You will need a bottle of MMS (the 22.4% sodium chlorite solution) and a bottle of activator. You can choose between citric acid, hydrochloric acid, and tartaric acid.

Sodium chlorite solutions are available in technical grade for industrial use and for water sterilisation, for example in swimming pools or drinking-water.

Every form of sodium chlorite used in laboratories and for water sterilisation is suitable for producing MMS. All sodium chlorite solutions that fulfil at least the purity criteria in Article 11 of the German Drinking Water Ordinance DIN EN 938 of 2009 are of excellent quality.

Most companies that sell MMS hold a considerable range: the standard bottles of 100ml or 120ml, bulk-buy discounts, and so forth. Jim Humble would buy sodium chlorite wherever he could acquire it cheaply, or wherever he could get his hands on it at all, for example swimming pool supplies. He was satisfied with its effect, and that it was well tolerated in Africa and South America by many to whom he gave it. Many sodium chlorite solutions of this quality that are on sale worldwide are produced for swimming pool hygiene. The situation is different in Europe. Due to poor nutrition and unnatural lifestyles on this continent, people here are often more sensitive, and react adversely in greater numbers, to even small quantities of impurities. If you are a rather sensitive person it would be safer for you to buy MMS of a higher quality. *High-quality MMS*

It is important that you set aside time to choose, prepare, and eat food that is as natural as possible.

Not all producers of MMS declare the purity grade of their solutions. If you prefer to take MMS that fulfils the conditions of the German Drinking Water Ordinance then ask the producer. For most users worldwide it is not of great importance what kind of MMS they take, but for some sensitive people it is.

Sodium chlorite solution of a purer quality, at 22.4 or 22.5%, is equal to a 28% sodium chlorite solution of a technical grade quality because the usual 20% additives resulting from the manufacturing process is omitted. *22.5% sodium chlorite solution*

For safety reasons and to minimise potential impurities, I prefer MMS that meets the purity criteria of Article 11 of the German Drinking Water Ordinance. I also prefer a 50% tartaric acid or a 3–5% hydrochloric acid as a 1:1 activator, and these should all be stored in glass or PE bottles. PET bottles are not suitable. *Protection in dark glass bottles*

Because of the legal situation in Germany, companies that sell MMS are not allowed to offer advice on the internal use of MMS. So do not be surprised if you find that most companies refuse to give you information on how to take MMS and at what dose.

If you read this book carefully you will find the answers to most of your questions.

If in future you find no results when using the search term 'MMS' on the internet, search under 'drinking-water steriliser', or 'drinking-water *Alternative search terms* purification agent', or for '22.5% sodium chlorite solution' and a suitable activator to produce chlorine dioxide, such as hydrochloric acid or tartaric acid, or alternatively search for '0.29% chlorine dioxide solution'.

MMS energy globules are another alternative for those interested in energy medicine. See chapter 8.15.

www.informierteGlobuli.de

Activator	Mix ratio	Number of drops	Activation time
Citric* / tartaric acid 5%	1:10	10 drops	3 minutes
Citric* / tartaric acid 10	1:5	5 drops	3 minutes
3–5% hydrochloric acid 50% tartaric acid or 50% citric acid*	1:1	1 drops	40–60 seconds

* Citric acid is only recommended as an activator if you cannot get hold of hydrochloric acid or tartaric acid.

In each case, the table refers to 1 drop of sodium chlorite solution and the appropriate mix ratio for the activators currently available. The activation time varies between 40 seconds and 3 minutes. You will recognise the activated solution by its gold-brown colour.

By the time the Fifth Edition of the *MMS Handbook* went to press, some retailers had ceased to sell MMS having come under pressure from the authorities to do so. In my opinion there is no rational reason for banning MMS. See chapter 17 'Legal Aspects'.

If that is possible, I recommend stocking up with plenty of MMS. It can be stored for many years in glass or PE bottles.

Your input is essential As things stand, you will have to campaign if you want MMS to continue to be freely available.

How to use MMS

To repeat once again at the outset: you use MMS on your own responsibility.

As a water purifier, it has not been approved for internal use. Therefore, as a doctor, I cannot advise you to use it for any purpose other than to sterilise water. But I do not see why I should be warning you against using it since many people have taken MMS and are grateful for the results they have seen. So with that I leave it to you to decide whether you want to conduct an experiment on yourself using MMS or not. However, if you have any serious ongoing complaints I advise you first and foremost to seek a medical explanation for the cause. A thorough diagnosis should be made before any treatment begins.

If you do decide to use MMS, please read this chapter very carefully. It is important to abide by Jim Humble's dosage instructions if you want good results. It is also important to observe the safety precautions: you are handling a hazardous substance.

Just as with any other highly effective tool, for example a lighter, cleaning agents etc., it should be used with the appropriate care, and it should be stored out of the reach of children and protected from direct sunlight. Before you buy or use it, please read the safety instructions thoroughly (chapter 11).

What you need

MMS is a 22.4% to 28% sodium chlorite solution that is activated with an acid. So you will need a bottle of MMS and a bottle of activator. Chapter 5 explains where to acquire it. You will need a clean, dry glass. Always use a glass, china or plastic cup: never use a metal container. It is not necessary to stir the solution, but if you so wish you can stir it using a wooden stirrer or a plastic spoon – no metal spoons should be used because some of the oxidative power would then be needlessly lost.

There are three ways of using MMS, all of which have been tested countless times: Jim Humble's new standard protocol, Jim Humble's

old standard protocol, and Clara's 6+6 protocol. All three ways are based on the same principle:
a 22.4% to 28% sodium chlorite solution is activated using diluted hydrochloric acid, tartaric acid or, if no other option is available, citric acid. After a certain time, water is added and the mixture is drunk. The individual protocols differ only in the number of drops, and the period of time that elapses between taking the doses. Jim Humble categorically recommends his new protocol to those who are critically ill. By administering lower doses of MMS regularly, users can take a higher total of drops per day than was possible by following the old protocol.

The following applies to all three above protocols:

6.1 Preparing and taking MMS

1. Put one drop of MMS in a clean, dry glass (free of washing-up liquid residues).

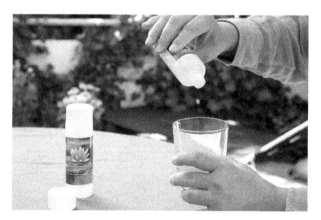

2. Add the activator.
   Drop ratio 1:1 with these activators:
   - 3–5% hydrochloric acid or
   - 50% tartaric acid or
   - 50% citric acid (only recommended under certain circumstances)

   This means you add one drop if using one of these activators. Ensure that the drops combine.

Preparing and taking MMS

Drop ratio 1:5 with these activators:
- 10% tartaric acid or
- pure, freshly-squeezed lime or lemon juice or
- 10% citric acid (only recommended under certain circumstances)

That means you add five drops if using one of these activators.

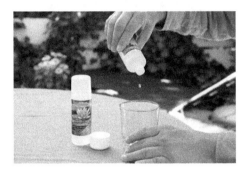

3. Swirl the glass.

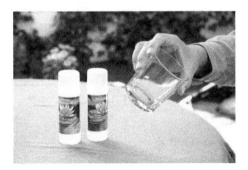

4. Wait for the activation time to pass.

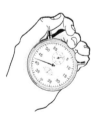

40–60 seconds with these activators:
- 3–5% hydrochloric acid or
- 50% tartaric acid or
- 50% citric acid (only recommended under certain circumstances)

3 minutes with these activators:
- 10% tartaric acid or
- pure, freshly-squeezed lime or lemon juice or
- 10% citric acid (only recommended under certain circumstances)

The solution turns yellow or gold-brown. This is how you know the drops have activated successfully: the active substance, chlorine dioxide, is formed – a gas that smells like chlorine.

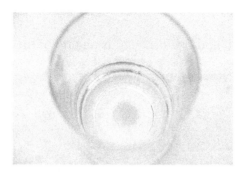

5. Top up the glass with 150–300ml of water; the water becomes a light yellow-green.

6. Drink the content of the glass on your own responsibility.

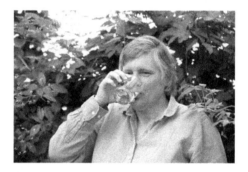

Always start at the lowest dose, and only increase the dose slowly and in accordance with your level of sensitivity if you tolerated the previous dose without any problems.

If you are using 3–5% hydrochloric acid, 50% tartaric acid, or (when no other option is available) 50% citric acid as an activator, add exactly the same number of drops of hydrochloric acid, tartaric acid or citric acid to the glass as you did of MMS. That is also the case with 50% citric acid. If you are using 10% citric acid as an activator, you need five times as much. Note the activation times, which are different for the various activators. With 10% citric acid or fresh lemon juice, the activation time is 3 minutes; with 50% tartaric acid, 3–5% hydrochloric acid, or 50% citric acid, it is only 40–60 seconds. Some producers note in their instructions that you only need an activation time of 20–30 seconds for 3–5% hydrochloric acid, 50% citric acid, or 50% tartaric acid. That is also Jim Humble's recommendation. My tests have shown that it is better to wait at least 40 seconds, even when using 5% hydrochloric acid. It is not, however, advisable to wait longer than 60 seconds. You can still use the mixture after up to two minutes, but after that, according to the experiential data known to me, you should throw it away. After more than two minutes it has activated too much. If you are using fresh lemon juice or a 10% citric acid solution, the optimal activation time is three minutes: in this case, a few seconds more or less is not of critical importance. It sometimes happens that something comes up unexpectedly and you cannot keep to the precise time. You can still use the mixture without problems after up to five minutes. After that it is better to throw it away and start again. If left to stand for a while, the MMS–acid mixture crystallises, no matter which activator is used. That is a perfectly normal process and does not mean that the MMS or the activator was of poor quality.

You should, however, throw it away then, and not use it. The majority of the chlorine dioxide released by the activator has by then escaped as a gas. By adding water at the right time, the chlorine dioxide dissolves in the water and can be used for up to four days as long as the solution is stored in a sealed container in a cool, dark place.

When you use MMS for the first time, the safest thing to do is to start with one drop so that you slowly begin to get a feel for it, and in order to avoid adverse reactions.

The best time to take it for most users is about 50–60 minutes after a meal, especially if you have a sensitive stomach. It has a more intense effect on an empty stomach but it can, under some circumstances, lead to symptoms of irritation. About 21% of users (according to my kinesiology tests) tolerate MMS better on an empty stomach; for about 20% (kinesiologically tested) it makes no difference; and for the remaining 59% it is, according to my kinesiology tests, better to take MMS 50–60 minutes after a meal.

No matter which activator you use it could be that the taste – whether right from the start or after some time – is not to your liking. If you feel nauseous, it might be that the smell of chlorine gas intensifies this memory, sparking an aversion. It would be a shame if you had to stop taking MMS as a result because there are some simple solutions to these problems. During the activation time it is wise to keep your nose two or three meters away from the MMS–activator mixture and you may want to open a window. Or put something such as a saucer over the glass to cover it – never use your hand. In addition, you could hold your nose closed while you drink the mixture. If you don't like the taste half-fill the glass with water and top it up with something you like the taste of. Use any juice **except** orange juice or juices with added vitamin C. You should also avoid nectars, fruit juice concentrates, and juice blends that contain thick puree.

Afterwards you could suck a sweet, but one that does not contain added vitamin C.

Vitamin C neutralises the effect of MMS **Vitamin C reacts with chlorine dioxide, thereby neutralising the effect of MMS.** Because of this, you should not take any vitamin C tablets four hours before or after taking MMS. The following juices (all without vitamin C) have proved to be very helpful in improving the taste of the mixture: apple, pineapple, cherry, cranberry, grape. Even though these juices contain high levels of vitamin C, we have not been able to detect a significant reduction in the effect of MMS.

Prepare the solution in the way you find it tastes best. It is also possible to increase the juice ratio to two-thirds. That slows down the effect somewhat but is not critical in the long term. Doing what feels right for you is always the best decision. If you heed these suggestions, it will be of great benefit to your process of recovery. Moreover, spending a few days feeling nauseous is not hugely conducive to health. You can be happy knowing that the MMS is working for you, but you can reach the same goal without experiencing strong reactions, even if that takes slightly longer. If you do experience nausea, diarrhoea, or serious flatulence, there is no cause for alarm. The complaints will completely abate within a few hours of discontinuing the MMS; in rare cases it may take a day or two. People usually feel very well afterwards (that is, of course, dependent on the general condition of your health, or on the underlying disease).

Digestive system reactions occur in most cases because of an intolerance to the activating acid. Citric acid, especially, can have an adverse effect. Complaints arise more frequently when the liver is in poor condition. You will find tips for such cases in chapter 7 'What to do if adverse reactions occur'. Alternatively, you have the option of switching to CDS, which does not need an activator, and which is almost universally well tolerated. You can also try MMS energy globules. See chapter 8.14.

Drink plenty of water You should drink plenty of water while you are on the MMS protocol. A person weighing 70kg should drink about 2.5 litres of water to aid elimination.

Increase the dose of MMS daily, starting with one drop and increasing to a maximum of 3 drops 8 times a day. Those are the general guidelines for people weighing up to 68kg. People who weigh more than 68kg should take correspondingly greater quantities, up to 4 (or even a maximum of 5) drops 8 times a day (when we say one drop, we always mean one drop of MMS plus the corresponding number of activator drops, plus activation time, plus water). It is important that you try to determine how many drops you personally can tolerate well. The best way to do this is to slowly increase and then pause or reduce if and when your body feels overstrained. If, at any time, you react with serious flatulence, diarrhoea or nausea, take a break until the complaints have abated. That will usually be within a few hours, or after a day or two. Then take two drops fewer than you did at the last dose. If that works well, stay at your personal maximum dose for a while (for about 14 days on average), then try to increase the dose carefully. If you become nauseous again, reduce even further, as described above, and increase later. Give your body only so much to process as it is able to tolerate. If you are not suffering from a life-threatening illness there is no urgency. If you are seriously ill, you should seek the supervision of a holistic doctor, alternative practitioner, and in some cases a psychotherapist.

It may also be wise for you to take MMS as a supplementary medication. Jim Humble recommends various approaches to taking MMS depending on the illness. You will find these approaches in chapter 12 'Dosage recommendations for patients with various illnesses'. Here are further basic principles for the use of MMS:

MMS is activated using 3–5% hydrochloric acid, or 50% tartaric acid or, if no other option is available, 50% citric acid:

Example of use 1

1. Put one drop of MMS into a clean, dry glass and add one drop of 3–5% hydrochloric acid or 50% tartaric acid. Swirl the glass to mix the drops.
2. Wait for the activation time of 40–60 seconds to pass. The drops turn a yellow or gold-brown colour; you can smell chlorine.
3. Top up the mixture with water and add juice to taste. Use any juice except orange juice and juices with added vitamin C.
4. Drink the activated mixture.

Repeat these steps 12 hours later, but increase the number of drops to two if you tolerated the first dose well. So you add two drops of 3–5% hydrochloric acid or 50% tartaric acid to two drops of MMS, wait for 40–60 seconds, fill the glass with water and juice, and then drink the mixture. The next time, you take three drops of MMS and three drops of 3–5% hydrochloric acid or 50% tartaric acid, then four of each and so on, as long as you can tolerate it well.

Information

If you can **easily tolerate** the dose of three drops of MMS eight times daily, take it until your complaints have completely disappeared. How long that takes depends on the illness. Then discontinue use, or reduce to a maintenance dose; see chapter 13 'MMS for healthy people'. Some users recommend taking a break of three or four weeks after taking MMS for three or four weeks, depending on your condition, because oxidative work can be strenuous for your body. If you notice that you become exhausted from taking MMS, it is better to take a break. During this time you should take plenty of vitamin C, other antioxidants and nutrients so that your organism is optimally supported. We have seen users who have taken six drops of MMS continuously for a year or more without experiencing problems of any kind. Quite the opposite, in fact: these people felt extraordinarily well and less susceptible to infections than before.

Example of use 2

MMS activated using 10% citric acid or freshly-squeezed lime or lemon juice*:

1. Put one drop of MMS into a clean, dry glass and add five drops of citric acid. Swirl the glass to mix the drops.
2. Wait for the activation time of three minutes to pass. The drops turn a yellow colour; you can smell chlorine.
3. Finally, top up the mixture with water, and then drink it; if desired add juice to taste (no orange juice, and no juices with added vitamin C).

* Citric acid is only recommended as an activator if you cannot get hold of hydrochloric acid or tartaric acid.

6.2 Acid–Alkaline Balance

The human body maintains an acid–alkaline balance at a blood pH-level of about 7.4. The pH-level is a dimensionless figure that describes the hydrogen ion activity in a liquid solution, thereby indicating whether a liquid solution exhibits an acidic or alkaline reaction. At a pH-level of 7, the solution is neutral; if the level is below 7 it is acidic; and if the value is above 7 it is alkaline (= basic).

pH-levels

The human body cannot tolerate large deviations – life is dependent on blood pH-values remaining between 7.0 and 7.8.

The human body ensures that the blood pH-value remains constant by using various buffers. Buffer acids and buffer bases are deployed as required, allowing a finely-tuned process of regulation to take place in a healthy body.

Due to unhealthy diets and stressful lifestyles many people, especially the chronically ill, have hyperacidic body tissue. It is therefore, in my opinion, a good idea for many people to use a lower dose of the activating acid. This is because the acid present in the body will be used as an activator in the reaction, to correspond to the reduced quantity of acid used. This measure will help neutralise the body if hyperacidity is an issue.

Hyperacidity of tissue in the chronically ill

MMS activation using reduced quantities of various acids:
- on 1 drop of MMS, **half a drop** of 3–5% of hydrochloric acid; or
- on 1 drop of MMS, **half a drop** of 50% tartaric acid; or
- on 1 drop of MMS, **half a drop** of 50% citric acid (only recommended under certain circumstances); or
- on 1 drop of MMS, **2 drops** of 10% citric acid or fresh lemon juice (instead of 5 drops)

Dosage suggestion

You can easily calculate the quantity of activator required for your dose of MMS. If you can only tolerate one drop of MMS, activate two drops of MMS, fill the glass with water, and throw away one-half.

Example of practical application for a single dose:
- on 2 drops of MMS, 1 drop of 3–5% hydrochloric acid
- on 2 drops of MMS, 1 drop of 50% tartaric acid

- on 2 drops of MMS, 4 drops of 10% citric acid or fresh lemon juice (only recommended under certain circumstances)

Example of practical application for a total daily quantity in eight doses:
- 24 drops of MMS with 12 drops of 3–5% hydrochloric acid
- 24 drops of MMS with 12 drops of 50% tartaric acid
- 24 drops of MMS with 48 drops of 10% citric acid or fresh lemon juice (only recommended under certain circumstances)

Try this to see whether it suits you better than Jim Humble's standard quantity of activator. Every individual is different. According to tests I have conducted, four out of five chronically ill patients react better to the reduced dose of activator acid described above.

User tip: measuring pH-value

You can determine the pH-value of urine using pH measuring strips. A pH-value of 7.0 is neutral. If the value of the urine sample is higher, it means it is alkaline (basic), meaning that the body is eliminating excess alkaline via the urine. If the value of the urine is below 7.0, the urine is acidic, meaning that excess acids are being eliminated via the urine. Normally, the pH-value of urine should move from the acidic range to the basic range within a period of 24 hours. If the pH-value of your urine is only ever in the acidic range (i.e. always < 7), you are certainly hyperacidic. If you want to measure this yourself, ensure that the pH-value can be clearly distinguished to one-tenth of an unit when buying the measuring strips.

If you test your urine for two or three days, you will know your condition. It is worth making a note of the values so that you can measure your progress.

6.2.1 Adding sodium bicarbonate to neutralise, stabilise and improve the taste

By adding sodium bicarbonate, the activated solution, topped up with water, can be moved back into the less acidic range. That has two effects:

Adding sodium bicarbonate

1. The solution becomes more stable and can, if necessary, be stored for longer without a significant diminishing of the chlorine dioxide content.
2. For many, the solution tastes better since most people find the taste of slightly acidic solutions pleasant, but find strongly acidic tastes unpalatable.

To acquire the quantity of chlorine dioxide that you want to produce by activating a certain number of drops, the dosage of sodium bicarbonate should follow the pattern below:

Sodium bicarbonate dose

after completing the activation and adding water, add eight equal-sized drops of a 10% sodium bicarbonate solution (use an empty, well-rinsed MMS bottle, shake before use to dissolve the sodium bicarbonate) for each drop of MMS. You can make a 10% sodium bicarbonate solution by dissolving a level teaspoon of sodium bicarbonate in nine teaspoons of water.

Alternatively, simply add 50mg of sodium bicarbonate to your day's ration of 24 activated MMS drops in a 0.75 or 1-litre bottle. 50mg is equal to the tip of a knife (see the image below).

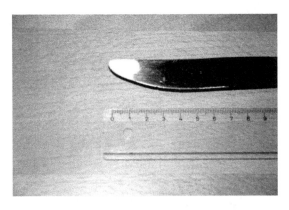

A knife-tip of sodium bicarbonate

If you are unsure, it is better to take too little sodium bicarbonate than too much. Upward deviations of 10% do no harm but if you mix in too much sodium bicarbonate, chlorine dioxide is used to form CO_2 and is no longer available for oxidation processes. Furthermore, when chlorine dioxide dissociates, sodium chlorate is formed in addition to the sodium chlorite; the former is generally not desirable in the body. You should not therefore exceed the stated quantities of sodium bicarbonate. When

6 • *How to use MMS*

taking a smaller dose of MMS, take correspondingly less sodium bicarbonate. If you only take a few drops of MMS, it is safer to add eight drops of a 10% sodium bicarbonate solution per drop of MMS.

If you do not want to produce a 10% sodium bicarbonate solution, you could alternatively add a small pinch of sodium bicarbonate for every 6 drops of 1:1 activated MMS in 250ml water at the end.

It is important that you only add the sodium bicarbonate after the activation of the MMS is complete, and after you have added the water or juice.

6.3 THE NEW STANDARD PROTOCOL: MMS 1000 PROTOCOL

For some time now, Jim Humble has been recommending filling a 1 to 1.5-litre bottle in the mornings with activated, ready-to-drink MMS, and marking the bottle on the outside into eight separate and equal units.

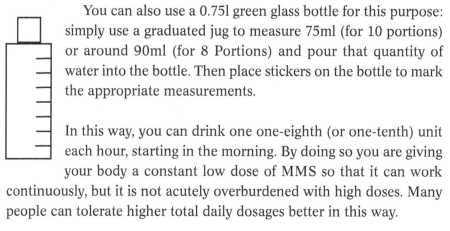

You can also use a 0.75l green glass bottle for this purpose: simply use a graduated jug to measure 75ml (for 10 portions) or around 90ml (for 8 Portions) and pour that quantity of water into the bottle. Then place stickers on the bottle to mark the appropriate measurements.

In this way, you can drink one one-eighth (or one-tenth) unit each hour, starting in the morning. By doing so you are giving your body a constant low dose of MMS so that it can work continuously, but it is not acutely overburdened with high doses. Many people can tolerate higher total daily dosages better in this way.

User tips on marking a glass bottle

- Take a clean glass bottle (0.75l, 1l or 1.5l).
- Mark seven lines on the outside of the bottle to make eight equal units, or nine lines to make ten equal units.
- Activate the desired number of MMS drops in a clean, dry glass.
- Top up the glass with water.
- Pour the mixture into the bottle, and top up with water and juice according to your taste until the bottle is full.
- Close the lid tightly.

Pour 125ml of water into a measuring jug and then pour this into the 1-litre bottle. Put a mark on the bottle at the point where the surface of the water reaches. Repeat seven times so that your bottle is correctly divided into eight units.   *User tip*
- Now empty the bottle. Activate the desired number of drops in a glass and top up with water. Then use a funnel to pour the mixture into the marked bottle and top the bottle up with water.
- You now have a ready-to-drink mixture with eight portions to consume at home or when you're on the road.

If you are away from home for a few days or if, for any reason, you do not wish to activate the MMS, top up the MMS with water only. If you want to add juice to improve the taste, add it to the glass directly before you drink it. Experience shows that it will then remain effective for at least three days, so long as the bottle is kept in a cool and dark place.   *User tip*

(If you add juice to the bottle, part of the acid as well as the vitamin C in the juice slowly but continuously reacts with the sodium chlorite, thereby reducing the original strength of the MMS mixture. You can still mix the 125ml of activated MMS solution with juice in a glass before drinking, to improve the taste.)

It is, of course, advisable to start slowly and cautiously with the 'MMS 1000 protocol', for example by taking three drops of MMS per day, or even less in difficult cases. The aim is to reach a dose of 24 drops of activated MMS, divided into eight units that are drunk hourly. If you are among those who show improvement on just a small dose of MMS then it is, of course, fine to remain on that low dose. The important thing is that you feel well, and it makes sense for individual people to take different doses. It is not a matter of ambitiously striving to reach a particular number of drops, or to break any records. The recommended doses are stated because they have worked well in the past, and so that you can profit from the experiences of others.

These are the average levels that have proved beneficial to adults weighing up to 68kg. People weighing more need correspondingly higher doses. Jim Humble recommends that adults weighing more than 68kg take up to 4 to 5 drops eight times a day. These are general guidelines; lower doses may be suitable in individual cases. For children, Jim Humble recommends a maximum single dose of 1 drop per 11.4kg of body weight. The maximum total daily amount for children depends on the severity of the illness and on the child's tolerance level. The guiding principle here is: as much as is necessary to bring about healing, as little as possible to avoid adverse reactions, just the same as for adults.

First and foremost take care not to do harm. There is no sense in giving high doses if it causes discomfort, severe diarrhoea or nausea. If adverse reactions occur, wait until they have abated, then restart on a dose two drops lower than previously. Overtaxing the human organism brings no benefits. If there is no life-threatening illness, you can proceed slowly and still reach your goal more quickly.

If you are able to maintain your reference dose for a week after the symptoms of illness have abated, the body will usually be free of harmful microorganisms and heavy metals.

6.4 JIM HUMBLE'S FORMER STANDARD PROTOCOL

In the past, Jim Humble tried to reach doses of 15 drops twice a day plus the respective quantity of activator to treat illnesses because that has proved in many cases to be an effective dose for adults weighing up to 68kg. It is essential that you first read the whole chapter before preparing any mixtures. In Europe, many people are incapable of tolerating such high doses from the outset without suffering nausea. This means you should gradually increase the dose if you want to avoid adverse reactions. If you take time to spread the dose over the course of a day, taking 3 drops per hour for eight hours, you have the advantage of a continuous saturation of chlorine dioxide over a long period of time. This approach allows many people to tolerate a higher total daily dose. That is why we prefer the new standard protocol.

Jim Humble also recommends another way in which relatively healthy people may administer MMS:

6.5 CLARA'S 6+6 PROTOCOL

This protocol is named after Clara Beltrones who has used it with great success on herself and others. Read the detailed case histories in Jim Humble's book *Breakthrough*, and see Clara Beltrones telling her story in the film *Understanding MMS*.

This protocol is suitable for people who suffer from illnesses that are generally regarded to be curable such as colds, flu-like infections, pains etc.

Jim Humble prefers small doses eight times a day every hour, as described in the new standard protocol, for bedridden patients and those with serious illnesses regarded as incurable.

Clara puts six drops of activated MMS in a glass of water with juice and waits for an hour to see how the patient fares.

If they are able to tolerate the six drops, she has the patient prepare a dose themselves an hour later, to ensure that they know how to prepare MMS. The patient remains there for a while following the second dose. If it has done them some good they can repeat that for a few days until they are healthy again. However, on the following day they should increase to 7+7 and so on, until they have reached 15+15. Two doses of 15 drops is the target dose for an adult weighing 68kg. I have already given extensive details on this above.

6.6 MMS for pregnant women

According to Jim Humble, pregnant women can take six drops of MMS preventively, but only if no adverse reactions occur.

Until now no harm to either the mother or baby has been observed. I think that that would be unlikely since no harmful by-products have been detected after using MMS, in contrast to many medications. Of course, a well-tolerated dose should be arrived at by slowly increasing the number of drops. Should the woman become ill during pregnancy, it would be wise to increase the dose of MMS accordingly. Depending on each individual instance, Humble recommends either following the new standard protocol, or the special dosage recommendation for the particular illness. According to Jim Humble, a large percentage of pregnant women suffering from malaria and other illnesses were cured with MMS at a missionary hospital in Kenya, where doctors too use MMS.

6.7 MMS for infants

Jim Humble has been recommending MMS for infants from the very beginning and – he reports – with great success. Babies usually tolerate a dose of one activated drop. Mix it with water and baby tea once the activation period is over, and administer it in a baby's bottle. Follow one of the protocols according to the type and severity of the illness, and bear in mind the limit of one drop per 11.4kg body weight per hour as a maximum starting dose. One drop of activated MMS will normally be fine. To be on the safe side you could start with half a drop, and then increase to one drop if your baby tolerates that well. You could activate four drops in the morning and give one-eighth of that each hour. If you activate four drops of MMS and top it up with 200ml of water and baby tea, give your baby 25ml eight times a day (about every hour), which is the equivalent of half a drop of activated MMS eight times. It is not critical if your baby wants to drink more or less at any given time. Go with what your baby takes. If, at the end of the day, the bottle with 200ml of activated MMS is empty, then the target has been reached. Bear in mind here individual tolerance.

If your baby does not drink much, you could dilute the four drops in 100ml of water, or less. If you notice that taking only four drops is not having the desired effect, you could try increasing the dose until your baby's health improves, but of course only increase by as much as your baby can tolerate.

Premature births
You can calculate an appropriate single dose for a significantly underweight premature baby by adding 0.1 of a drop per 11.4kg of body weight. Don't worry too much about each decimal point here. If in doubt, start with less: you can always increase the dose later. If you want to give 0.1 of a drop, activate one drop, wait for the activation period to pass, and top up a baby bottle with water and baby tea (juice only from the third or fourth month, if the infant tolerates juice). You can now give the baby one-tenth of this mixture, ideally spread over a day in ten doses every hour or two. This is the safest method for prematurely born babies, and for infants in their first months. You can then increase the dose as required.

Follow this approach to calculate and prepare various quantities of MMS. Activated MMS solution stored in a closed container in the refrigerator will maintain its potency for three days, usually even four. After that it will have lost its oxidising power and should not be used.

If you search for the term 'malaria baby' on YouTube, you will find a video which features a baby that was treated in a missionary hospital in Kenya in 2004. This baby's fever reached 40 °C. Two hours after being given MMS, the temperature had fallen to 38.3 °C.

Jim Humble has also been successful in administering MMS externally on babies' skin, and has never observed intolerance reactions while

6.8 MMS for children

Observe the safety instructions, and store the MMS and the activator out of the reach of children. It is best to put it away immediately after preparing it for your child.

Observe safety instructions

Children and teenagers can enjoy the benefits of MMS just like everyone else. Of course, the same problems – flatulence, watery stools, diarrhoea and nausea – can occur. It is very difficult to do anything once an aversion to the taste or smell has developed. It is therefore especially important with children to begin slowly with one drop of activated MMS and to have plenty of juice at hand. Do not allow your child to sniff at the glass during the activation period. Prepare the drink with water and juice and tell your child to drink it quickly so that they don't taste and smell it for too long. If necessary, give them another glass of pure juice afterwards. The unpleasant taste is amplified by waiting and breathing. It is best to drink the glass of MMS in one single attempt, and then immediately drink some pure juice. The child can then enjoy the juice in peace.

> When up to three drops of MMS are mixed with oatmilk, it is almost impossible to taste the chlorine dioxide. This is, therefore, a good way of giving MMS to children, and the efficacy of MMS in oatmilk has been proven repeatedly.

User tip: oatmilk

If you are finding it impossible to persuade your child to drink the MMS solution, you could put the activated MMS in a vegetable cellulose capsule, to be swallowed with water. However, this is quite laborious. It can also lead to various complications, especially if your child is reluctant to swallow the capsules. On no account should you try to make your child swallow capsules against their will. The best way of getting the activated MMS into the capsules is as follows:

acquire some vegetable capsules, a syringe and a cannula. Activate the MMS and dilute in two teaspoons of water. Draw up into the syringe and inject into one half-capsule. Using the other half, seal the capsule. You will need a number of capsules to administer the desired dose.

Make absolutely sure beforehand that your child is able to swallow capsules. Try that in advance using an empty capsule or a capsule filled with water. Have a large glass of water at the ready.

It is much easier in the long run if you can persuade your child to drink the solution. After taking MMS a few times, children usually notice that it is doing them good and they want to take it. Observe the maximum starting dose for children: one drop per 11.4kg body weight per hour. That means that if you have a child weighing 11kg, you can activate eight drops in the morning, mix with water and juice, and give one-eighth of this every hour. If your child weighs 6kg, activate four drops in the morning and give one-eighth of this each hour. You can calculate the appropriate dose for your child's weight accordingly. If your child tolerates this dose well, and you notice only a slight improvement in condition, increase the dose. A paediatric clinic discovered that it was beneficial for children under three who did not improve at the standard dose, to take one drop per 3kg of body weight twice daily, or alternatively, if it was better tolerated, the same dose spread over the whole day. If your child becomes nauseous or has diarrhoea you should stop or reduce the dose.

6.9 SLOW ACTIVATION BASED ON THE FISCHER METHOD

Dr Hartmut Fischer has developed an almost tasteless chlorine dioxide solution by using the following procedure.

In the evening put 100–200ml of tap water in a clean 1-litre bottle. Add the desired number of drops of MMS ($NaClO_2$ solution) and swirl to mix. Add the appropriate number of drops of activator. Top up the bottle with water until full. Close the bottle tightly, swirl again, and store overnight in a cool, dark place.

The solution is ready to use on the following day and can be taken in eight to ten units spread over the course of the day. If desired, add sodium bicarbonate in the morning (a maximum of 50mg per 20 drops of MMS).

The sodium chlorite is slowly activated overnight, producing chlorine dioxide. The chlorine dioxide yield is considerably less than it would be using the quick activation method, but the quantity of chlorine dioxide is clearly enough to achieve an adequate therapeutic effect since Dr Fischer is satisfied with the effectiveness of his method. He usually takes

20 drops of MMS plus 20 drops of 4% hydrochloric acid as a daily ration. He adds a maximum of 50mg of sodium bicarbonate the following morning for those who dislike the taste. That corresponds roughly to a knife-tip.

Doing that stops the activation process. The solution is almost as tasteless as pure water and the solution will keep for a while. In extreme cases, you can still use the chlorine dioxide solution neutralised with sodium bicarbonate for up to three weeks without it decreasing in efficacy.

In addition, slow activation has the advantage that those who cannot stand drinking quickly-activated MMS, can now take MMS once more.

If you are among those who cannot bear to take MMS because of the taste, but would like to take it, then it is certainly worth trying this method. If you forget to make the preparation one evening you can still use the slow activation as long as you wait for at least three hours. That means you could activate a bottle slowly, using the Fischer method, and take your first dose from it three hours later. *Improving the taste*

However, the activation advances further and presumably also has a stronger effect if you allow the solution to stand overnight. Leaving the solution for longer is not a problem. Even if you forget it for a day or two and only then add the sodium bicarbonate, or if you use it on the third day, the solution is just as effective as it was after the first night because the activation proceeds slowly and the chlorine dioxide produced dissolves immediately in the water and cannot escape.

Slow activation according to Fischer is, with regard to the stability of the solution, very low maintenance. *Low maintenance*

There are hardly any problems with regard to tolerance. If reactions such as diarrhoea or nausea occur, indicating that the organs of elimination are overburdened, it is – as with all the other protocols – advisable to reduce the dose or to take a break altogether.

6.10 WHO SHOULD TAKE PARTICULAR CARE WHEN TAKING MMS?

Anyone who is sensitive to triggers of any kind should approach MMS with great care. This includes people who have severe allergies to various substances and anyone who has noticed that they do not tolerate various medications particularly well. I advise against taking MMS if you have an allergy to chlorine smells (e.g. triggered in swimming pools). There is *No MMS with chlorine allergy* no known experience that we can refer to regarding this. Anyone with a chlorine allergy taking MMS is experimenting on unfamiliar territory.

Patients who have been undergoing medical treatment for decades, taking a number of medications concurrently over long periods of time, should also take particular care when taking MMS. This is because MMS works as a detoxifier, giving the liver and kidneys more work to do.

Care with liver dysfunction People with liver dysfunction or liver diseases, or who suffer from renal insufficiency or who only have one kidney, should also be very careful with MMS. If they do decide to take MMS they should also simultaneously support the organs of elimination. CDS is preferable if the patient suffers from kidney or liver damage.

You should not take MMS without having read the whole book.

Particular care should also be taken by people who have suffered gas poisoning, or if family members have had traumatic experiences with gas poisoning.

Haemophiliacs

Patients who take Marcumar Haemophiliacs should take particular care with MMS, as should those people who take Marcumar or other blood-thinning medications. MMS works against the coagulation of red blood cells. That is normally beneficial to health but could lead to an overdose of the blood-thinning medications. It would be wise to have your INR values (previously known as Quick values) checked with your GP to avoid an increased risk of bleeding.

You should also stop taking MMS for 14 days before an operation for the same reason. This is not limited to internal use but to all kinds of use.

For those who want to take the burden off the liver and kidneys, it is probably helpful to start with foot baths, or full baths if you are able to tolerate it. This way the detoxification process happens largely via the skin; see chapter 7 ('What to do if adverse reactions occur') and chapter 8 ('More ways of administering MMS').

6.11 CONTRAINDICATIONS

Operations

Oxygen administration

Artificial respiration MMS use should be discontinued if the patient is being given additional oxygen or artificial respiration. Since chlorine dioxide is transported by the same part of the red blood cells as oxygen, the oxygen should be given priority in such cases. Other than that, the only contraindication known to me is an impending operation. MMS should be discontinued 14 days before an operation.

In individual cases abstention of a few days might be sufficient, but I find 14 days more satisfactory in order to be certain that there is no more blood thinning than is appropriate before undergoing an operation.

Allergies to sodium chloride or chlorine dioxide would also be further contraindications. However, I have never heard of such circumstances.

If an activator is not tolerated because of an allergy, especially when used externally, it is advisable to change the activator. It happens very rarely that citric acid leads to irritation of the skin when used externally due to the formation of sodium citrate or due to the high acid ratio. Changing to the 3–5% hydrochloric acid or tartaric acid remedies this. *Change activator*

No further contraindications are known to me.

Gold crowns, shrapnel, artificial hips etc. are not contraindications. I personally have a few gold crowns and, during my phase of testing and experimenting, I used MMS in various ways for over a year and have never encountered a problem with the crowns. *Gold crowns*

Meanwhile there have probably been millions of people who have taken MMS and there have been no reports of problems with metal implants in whatever form.

I suspect that this is due to the body's own intelligence in transporting the chlorine dioxide to exactly where it is needed for oxidation.

Taking high potency homeopathic medicine at the same time is not contraindicated in my opinion. I have not found that MMS interferes with classical homeopathic treatment. *Homeopathy*

Neither do you need to worry about your intestinal flora, or other good bacteria needed for the upkeep of physiological processes in the human body. I have not observed any adverse effect on digestive function even when used continuously over a long period of time. *Intestinal flora*

Your vitamin C levels are the only thing you need to monitor if taking MMS for periods of months. Eat one vitamin-rich meal every day, or plan vitamin C doses so that there is an interval of 4 hours between them and doses of MMS. *Vitamin C interval*

6.12 POSSIBLE RESPONSES TO MMS

1. You quickly become well. That will presumably make you very happy. If the symptoms disappear you can decide whether to discontinue use of MMS or to continue with a maintenance dose.

2. You slowly improve.
It is usually worth persevering. As long as the symptoms are receding you are on the right track.
3. Some symptoms improve, others do not.
It would be wise to continue taking MMS if you tolerate it well. Depending on the severity and type of illness, DMSO or MMS 2 could be helpful as a supplement.
4. All your symptoms return.
If previous symptoms return, it probably means that your system is processing old toxic burdens. This basically means that your body is using MMS to take care of left-over stores of harmful residues, or of accumulations of previous illnesses you have gone through. The symptoms should disappear after a reasonable time. Homeopaths regard the following as a good guide to determine what a reasonable period is:

an organism needs the same number of months to recover from a chronic illness as the number of years the illness has persisted. That means that acute illnesses heal very quickly, whereas an illness that has existed for five years will take about five months to cure. An allergy that has existed for 20 years would, accordingly, need 20 months to clear completely. Fortunately, with MMS things move along much more quickly, at least when it comes to the elimination of symptoms. A homeopathic conception of a complete cure is a holistic process involving body, mind and spirit, and not just the elimination of symptoms.
5. You suffer from watery stools or slight diarrhoea.
That is a good sign. Your body is cleansing itself via the bowels. Do not increase the dose for the time being and you may want to consider reducing the dose a little if the diarrhoea becomes more severe. In most cases this cleansing phase is largely finished in 14 days and stools return to normal.
6. You suffer from severe flatulence, severe diarrhoea, nausea or vomiting. This happens when your body has more toxins to eliminate than it can handle.
It helps if you stop taking MMS and wait until you feel well again. When you restart, do so slowly on a reduced dose. If you find it impossible to tolerate even the smallest internal doses, you could use other means to detoxify your liver and use MMS only as a foot bath or, if possible, a full bath for the time being. You will find a complete

list of tips in chapter 7 'What to do if adverse reactions occur'. Reducing the level of acid by adding sodium bicarbonate, as described in chapters 6.2.1 and 6.9, can also be very helpful.

In some circumstances, you might need the support and supervision of a holistic doctor or alternative practitioner. You will also find a few things you can do to help yourself in the 'Guidelines for healthy living' (chapter 18).

7. MMS has no effect.

    This is very rare. You may not have reached the required dose for you, in which case increasing the dose further could help. If you observe absolutely no results whatsoever when taking a maximum total daily dose of 45 drops, MMS' oxidative ability to kill pathogens and eliminate heavy metals is not sufficient for healing. It is very likely that there are obstacles to healing present. I recommend you read chapter 18 'Guidelines for healthy living' thoroughly, eliminate fields of interference, and if necessary find a kinesiologist, psychotherapist or healer. Having said that, if you have a severe or protracted chronic condition, I assume that you are in the care of a doctor or alternative practitioner.

7

WHAT TO DO IF ADVERSE REACTIONS OCCUR

Jim Humble has never observed side effects in the true sense of the term. The only thing he has observed is the occurrence of flatulence, diarrhoea and nausea, caused by the toxic burden of the pathogens killed. At a dose of two drops, Jim Humble has only observed nausea in about 1 in 500 users. Diarrhoea is more common – it is part of the cleansing process and is sometimes unavoidable. As long as it is not excessive you do not need to do anything. If you have severe diarrhoea, discontinue use of MMS and take plenty of fluids with salt. It should be sufficient to drink one level teaspoon of prehistoric rock salt dissolved in water in the mornings and evenings. You can treat the diarrhoea with natural cures, homeopathic remedies and, if necessary, charcoal tablets. If it is more serious, consult your doctor or alternative practitioner. Start taking MMS again when you feel better, ideally taking two drops fewer than the dose at which problems arose.

Eat an apple   Eating an apple a quarter of an hour before taking MMS has proved useful as a way of preventing nausea. In many cases nausea only occurs at the start, sometimes only once, when you reach the threshold of nausea. As you continue, a higher dose can then generally be tolerated easily without nausea.

Drink more water   Severe nausea indicates that the organs of elimination are under pressure. If you drink fewer than three litres of water each day, drink more. Stop taking MMS for a while until you feel better. Then restart by taking two drops fewer than the dose that brought on the nausea. There are

Deacidification   many ways of cleansing the liver: artichoke juice, fumewort, milk thistle, deacidification with alkaline foods, alkaline baths, alkaline salts, or ho-

Seek advice from a homeopath or a holistic doctor or alternative practitioner   meopathic remedies such as Chelidonium, Nux Vomica, Lycopodium, to name but a few possible remedies. If you are not very familiar with homeopathy it is better to seek advice from a homeopath because homeopathy demands a very specific individual diagnosis, and success on an indication basis is very rare.

Chinese medicine, with acupuncture and herbs, can also be used to

What to do if adverse reactions occur

assist the liver. Seek advice from a holistic doctor or alternative practitioner in your area. There are many ways in which they can help you. It is also very helpful to eat a good diet; most importantly, follow a diet that is free from artificial flavourings and preservatives, and one which is as natural as possible, with plenty of fruit and vegetables. The single most important thing for a healthy liver, however, is a balanced temper. More on that in chapter 18 'Guidelines for healthy living'. *Plenty of fruit and vegetables*

If, even after repeated attempts, you still find it impossible to increase the MMS dose to more than two drops without becoming nauseous, there are a number of ways to proceed.

You could try taking the lower dose for a long period of time. If you feel slightly better after a couple of weeks, carry on at this level. Pathogens are certainly being killed and toxins eliminated.

Everyone is unique. It may be that your body works better at a slower but continuous pace than if you were to overburden it with high doses. I personally know two users who took doses of three drops over a long period of time with good effect. Others have had good results taking five or six drops.

You do not necessarily need 15 drops to reach your effective dose. Fifteen drops is the average effective dose and is only meant to serve as a point of orientation.

However, if you have been taking two drops for a long period of time and you observe no improvement in your condition and you cannot increase the dose, it is necessary to first undergo a thorough detoxification treatment, ideally under the supervision of an experienced holistic doctor or alternative practitioner in your area, so that your body is detoxified and purged sufficiently so that it can tolerate MMS at effective doses. *Detoxification treatment*

If your circulation is strong enough to cope with a 20 to 30-minute bath without problems, you could also add MMS to your bathwater. Jim Humble states on his website that people who could not tolerate more than seven drops orally could tolerate far more drops after taking a bath with MMS, without suffering nausea. More on this in chapter 8 'More ways of administering MMS'. A foot bath could also be helpful to you. *MMS baths*

Foot bath

If you take too much activated MMS by mistake, drink a large glass of water. If that is not enough, drink another glass of water with 1–5g vitamin C. If you don't have such large quantities of vitamin C at hand, a glass of water containing a level teaspoon of sodium bicarbonate is a good alternative, but decide on one or the other. *Antidote: 1–5g vitamin C or 1 tsp. sodium bicarbonate*

7 • What to do if adverse reactions occur

Drink water to bring about vomiting

According to Jim Humble, swallowing more than half a teaspoon of sodium chlorite solution does no harm other than causing terrible nausea. To avoid this, drink as much water as possible, ideally containing half a teaspoon of sodium bicarbonate per glass. If possible, drink enough to cause you to vomit.

If your child drinks a whole bottle, Jim Humble advises you to go to the emergency unit of the nearest hospital and tell the doctor that your child has drunk sodium chlorite solution.

There are people who cannot tolerate MMS on an empty stomach. If you have a sensitive stomach it is better to take MMS 50 to 60 minutes after a meal.

Avoid excess acid

Some people are only unable to tolerate the excess acid which results from using large quantities of citric acid. Switch to using tartaric acid or hydrochloric acid as an activator. After changing, many users who previously had problems were able to tolerate MMS well. It is also possible to improve the taste and neutralise the acid by adding sodium bicarbonate (see chapter 6.2.1).

Some users react to even the smallest quantity of impurities in technical grade MMS. It could be worth switching to MMS of a purer quality since it is more easily tolerated by many Europeans.

Blood thinning

One user wrote to me saying that MMS had had a strong blood-thinning effect. He regularly had his Quick values checked because he was taking Marcumar to thin his blood and he discovered that his blood had become thinner.

However, I do not consider this to be an adverse effect but rather a part of the healing process because it is certainly not healthy for people to be taking blood-thinning medication throughout their lives. No interaction with other medications has been observed so far. The emergence of an allergy cannot, of course, be ruled out because allergies can develop against any substance. That could happen when eating an apple or a slice of bread. I have never heard of anyone reacting allergically to MMS.

8

MORE WAYS OF ADMINISTERING MMS

There are a number of other ways of administering MMS apart from oral use.

8.1 SPRAYED ONTO THE SKIN

Protocol for skin spray

To prepare a skin spray you will need a clean, dry bottle with a volume of at least 60ml and a spray top. The glass bottles with a spray top that you can obtain from pharmacies are best. They don't react with the MMS. It is important that none of the materials in the plastic, such as the softening agents (plasticisers), are released. Even if you 'only' spray something onto your skin, the substance in question can be detected in the urine 30 minutes later. Taking MMS is meant to detoxify your body, not add to your toxic load.

Put 20 drops of MMS in the bottle and add the activator. When the activation period is over, top up the bottle with 60ml of water and close the spray top. Spray the MMS onto the area of skin that you wish to treat. Repeat this every hour or two. It can be a good idea to do this for a period of days, depending on the severity of the problem. After spraying the activated MMS leave it to dry. **Pure MMS (i.e. not activated)** *Burns* **should only ever be used to treat burns. Moisten the burned area with pure MMS, that is, a 22.4% sodium chlorite solution. You should then wash off the moistened area with water within 30–60 seconds without fail.** Otherwise you will only aggravate the condition instead of improving it. If you don't have any water to hand, any other drinkable fluid can be used as an alternative. This is a way of providing first aid for yourself or others in cases of first- to third-degree burns, if you wish to do so. In cases of third-degree burns it is imperative that you seek a doctor or go to the nearest hospital.

In all other cases simply leave the sprayed area as it is, or wash it off with water after three minutes, depending on your preference. However, you should always wash off the old, dried moisture before spraying the area anew.

Insect bites

Skin diseases

MMS as a deodorant

Jim Humble recommends using a spray on insect bites, warts, maculae or skin alterations, fungus infections, acne, skin diseases such as tinea (ringworm), atopic dermatitis, or psoriasis, inflammations, indeed any kind of skin problem, even skin cancer. We have also seen good results when treating wounds, even dog bites. MMS is also excellent as a deodorant.

In cases of skin diseases that affect a large area it is advisable to test first on a small area to see whether or not your skin tolerates MMS. The MMS spray should never be allowed to get into the eyes. That can cause irritations because the concentration is much higher for external application than it is for internal use.

The solution can be used for four days.

As a comparison: this is equivalent to about 40 drops of MMS in half a glass of water.

If the spray burns or irritates your skin too much, dilute the solution until it no longer burns. Throw away half the solution, top it up with water, and then try it again on a small area of skin. If it still burns, dilute it further until you can tolerate it. Jim Humble sprayed and rubbed in activated MMS onto his face every day for six months. He also rubbed it intensively into a few other sensitive areas of skin. After six months, the areas of skin treated were in excellent condition. The patches of skin that had been subjected to intense long-term spraying with MMS were just as soft and tender, if not even more so, than the areas left unsprayed. By now, Jim Humble has years of personal experience of externally applying MMS and has never observed any harm done to the skin.

According to Jim Humble all kinds of skin types have been sprayed with MMS, even baby skin, including new-born babies.

MMS, prepared according to Jim Humble's protocol, does not attack healthy cells. Do not place the bottle in direct sunlight. You can use the solution for up to four days if stored in a dark place at room temperature. After that, pour it away and prepare more if you need it.

Tip for those with green fingers

Here is another tip for those with green fingers:

MMS spray can be used on plants affected by mould growth.

8.2 BATHING WITH MMS

The skin is our largest organ – that is probably the reason why bathing with MMS is so effective.

One specific advantage is that the unpleasant taste is not a problem. Another benefit is that bathing with MMS can often raise people's nausea threshold.

> **Warning: do not bathe alone if you are frail, weak, or have circulation problems.** Ask someone to supervise as you bathe. This precaution has less to do with the MMS than it does with the fact that bathing in warm water can cause circulation failure in those who are frail, or who are predisposed to such problems. It is important to come out of the bath at the first sign of such a problem. If you know that you tend to have circulation problems when bathing, it is wise to run lukewarm water into the bath, topping up with warm water as required.

Tip

Protocol for use in a bath

a) The bathtub must be cleaned thoroughly. Ensure that it is perfectly clean, otherwise the chlorine dioxide will react with soap, chalk or dirt residues and become less effective. Clean the bathtub, rinse thoroughly with clean water, and dry with a clean, dry towel. If the towel still shows signs of dirt, repeat the cleaning process. *Clean bathtub*

b) As a starting dose, activate 20 drops of MMS using twice the usual quantity of activator. This means: *Twice the quantity of activator*
- for 20 drops of MMS you add 40 drops 3–5% hydrochloric acid. Then swirl the glass so that the drops mix, and wait for the 40–60 second activation period to pass before filling the glass with water.
- or for 20 drops of MMS you add 40 drops of 50% tartaric acid. Then swirl the glass so that the drops mix, and wait for the 40–60 second activation period to pass before filling the glass with water.
- or for 20 drops of MMS you add 40 drops of 50% citric acid. Then swirl the glass so that the drops mix, and wait for the 40–60 second activation period to pass before filling the glass with water.
- or for 20 drops of MMS you add 200 drops of 10% citric acid. Then swirl the glass so that the drops mix, and wait for the three

minute activation period to pass before filling the glass with water.

You should never drink this quantity of activated MMS.

MMS on open skin   It is important to start with less MMS if you have open wounds or deep wounds; Jim Humble recommends 16 drops. You know your individual level of sensitivity; you may want to start at an even lower level. When you take your next baths, slowly increase the dose to 40–60 drops or more. Test it to see for yourself what works for you.

No soap or artificial bathing additives   c) Put only water into the bathtub. You should not use soap or any other artificial bathing additives. Experienced users who like to experiment have discovered that adding a handful of Himalaya salt to a full tub has a pleasant effect and does not reduce the effect of MMS, possibly even increasing its effect. If you first take a few baths without adding Himalaya salt and then a few baths with it, you can find out for yourself what you prefer.

d) Pour the mixture containing the activated MMS into the bathwater. You have added double the quantity of activator so that the sodium chlorite is activated quickly and so that much chlorine dioxide is released. Stir the mixture in the water. The water is sterilised within seconds. It is not important how full the bath is. Fill it up to a level you are happy with and put your hand in to see if the temperature is to your liking.

e) Now get into the water. Make sure the water covers your whole body, and pour bathwater over the parts of your body that are above the waterline. You should wash all parts of your face with the bathwater.

Rub afflicted body parts   Depending on sensitivity, rub the solution into the afflicted body parts. It is no problem if some of the heavily-diluted MMS solution gets into the eyes: simply wipe it away. A ready-to-drink solution or the concentration in spray form can lead to irritations but the bathwater solution is too weak to cause any problems. Pour the water over your head and massage it into your scalp. Warning: this can turn the hair blond, depending on the concentration of chlorine dioxide and on how long you wait before rinsing it out. Run some hot water when the water has cooled somewhat: the heat opens the pores and helps the MMS to penetrate further into the tissue. You can come out of the bath after 30 minutes but you can stay for longer if you wish. Clean the bath again when you have finished bathing. If you suffer from a persistent skin problem, it might be a good idea to take a bath at appropriate, regular intervals.

In addition to people with skin problems, users with a particularly low nausea threshold have found MMS baths particularly beneficial. Many have been able to tolerate significantly more MMS orally even after only one bath. Jim Humble suspects that the pathogens killed and the toxic substances neutralised when bathing are eliminated directly via the skin. As a result they no longer circulate in the blood and do not place a strain on the liver, which would otherwise be responsible for their elimination. *Raises nausea threshold*

An MMS bath can eliminate pathogens and toxins located on or in the skin, in the subcutaneous fatty tissue, and even in the musculature below, depending on how far the MMS can penetrate and how many pathogens and toxins are present. This process relieves the pressure on the liver. It is of course worthwhile to increase the oral dose of MMS to an effective level as soon as it is possible to do so without jeopardising your well-being. If you are seriously ill, Jim Humble recommends continuing to take a daily oral dose, even as you are bathing in MMS.

8.3 Brushing teeth and mouth washing with MMS

Protocol for general mouth washing

Activate ten drops of MMS and top up with half a glass of water. *Protocol*

Pour the MMS solution over a soft toothbrush, brush the teeth carefully and massage the gums gently. Do this three or four times a day for the first four days, then once a day is enough. *Use a soft toothbrush*

You can use the rest of the solution to rinse your mouth and gargle with. If possible, keep the solution in the mouth for a few minutes so that the chlorine dioxide has time to penetrate into the oral mucosa. Then spit it all out. You can repeat the process if you still have some of the solution left over in the glass. Or you can use some of the solution to rinse the mouth and some to gargle with. Experience has shown that sensitive or raw areas on the tongue, gums, cheeks or roof of the mouth are not aggravated by this. Quite the contrary: bacteria and other pathogens are killed. Sensitive, raw or inflamed areas usually heal quickly using this method. Brushing teeth and rinsing with MMS at least once *Leave the solution in the mouth for a few minutes*

a day for a few weeks is usually enough for most users to re-establish good oral health. Brushing teeth and mouth washing with MMS two or three times a week is sufficient to maintain this condition.

Some people have reported that their toothaches have disappeared within minutes of swilling the mouth with activated MMS for two minutes. How long the absence of pain lasted varied; usually about 12–24 hours after one or two MMS treatments, repeating when necessary. It is important to brush the painful tooth directly so that the chlorine dioxide can reach the bacteria causing the problem.

Discolouration disappears and bad breath is reduced

People who have been regularly brushing their teeth with MMS report that discolouration gradually disappears and that the teeth become a lighter colour. MMS users have also had success in treating bad breath when they brush the backmost part of the tongue with MMS solution. Jim Humble advises brushing as far back as the brush will go because the bacteria that colonise the furthermost part of the tongue produce sulphur dioxide. When they disappear, so does the bad breath. Dental

Dental calculus

calculus that has existed for years will take longer to disappear if it is only treated with MMS. It is therefore advisable first to have a dentist remove the dental calculus, and then regularly brush the teeth with activated MMS as a prophylactic measure.

8.4 MMS ENEMAS

Just as with infusions, enemas can transport MMS into the blood plasma as well as into the red blood cells. That increases the effectiveness because MMS reaches areas via the blood plasma that the red blood cells cannot reach. Conducting an enema is, admittedly, slightly laborious, but it is possible to do so at home.

You will need

You will need the following: an irrigator (a container that can contain 1.5 litres of water), a rubber tube attached to the irrigator with a rounded cap, which ideally has a kind of valve on it so that you can regulate the water intake. If you don't have such a thing, you can order it at a health food shop or in some pharmacies. You will also need warm water and cooking salt.

You should conduct the first two or three enemas without MMS to free your bowels from faeces. If you have conducted a number of enemas, skip the following enema instructions.

Instructions for MMS enemas

Take off your clothes so that you can introduce the plastic catheter into your anus. It can be helpful to have a second person to assist you by filling and holding the irrigator, but it is possible to do it all yourself.

Put half a litre of hot water into the irrigator and add a teaspoon of salt. When the salt has dissolved, add as much hot and cold water as is needed to achieve body temperature. Open the valve on the catheter and let out the air from the tube. When the water comes through, test again to see whether it is at a comfortable temperature. Close the valve.

If necessary, lubricate or grease the plastic end sparingly.

Insert the plastic end slowly and carefully into the anus, open the valve and allow (for an average-sized adult) between 0.75 and 1 litre of water to flow into the bowel. Close the valve again. Pull the catheter slowly and carefully out of the anus. Squeeze the sphincter because the water causes a spontaneous desire to defecate. This desire passes after a while. Once the water has risen higher, the desire to defecate will return about 5 to 10 minutes later. You can then yield to this and defecate. If you yield immediately, the only thing that comes out is the water you put in. The salt is important so that your bowel does not 'drink' the water. Repeat the enema procedure two more times. If you have had multiple enemas over a number of consecutive days, repeating once is sufficent, making a total of two water flushes rather than three. Massaging the belly might help; try it to see what you find comfortable. If you find that you can only hold the water for a short while, simply do it one additional time, that is not a problem. It is much easier once you have some experience. It is important to ensure that the irrigator containing the water is held well above the level of the anus because the water flows down with gravity. If you have not put in enough water, there will not be enough pressure to get the water to flow into the bowel. So you could, for example, put 1.5 litres into the irrigator but only allow a maximum of 1 litre to flow into the bowel. You need to keep the irrigator at least at shoulder height, but at the same time keep an eye on the water level so that you can turn off the valve in time. This is why it is so much easier if you have someone to help you.

After three water enemas, each with a teaspoonful of cooking salt, you are ready for the MMS enema. Start with a low dose of MMS. If you have never taken MMS orally, start with one drop in the morning, then activate two drops in the evening. The next morning activate three drops, and four drops in the evening, until you reach a maximum of 15 drops, twice.

If you already have some experience of taking MMS orally, stay well below the nausea threshold when you start. Add plenty of water to the dose of activated MMS so that it can flow into the bowel. The best approach is to calculate double the dose of MMS and then leave half the water in the irrigator and throw it away afterwards, because not all the water will flow out due to the pressure ratios.

Half a litre of water is more than enough for an MMS enema when the bowel is already cleansed. I would therefore top up the activated MMS with a litre of water and then allow half that to flow into the bowel. If you prefer to use syringes, clysters or anything else, then 120ml of water will suffice. Now try to keep the mixture of activated MMS and water in your bowels for as long as you can so that as much chlorine dioxide as possible is absorbed through the intestinal walls. Of course, no cooking salt is used in the enema when MMS is used.

Take these enemas at least twice a day. If diarrhoea or nausea occur, take a break until the complaints abate. You can then restart with a reduced dose. Take care of yourself. Taking enemas at certain intervals, or when you have an acute infection, is a good idea because it helps to detoxify the body.

In our grandparents' time every home would have had the necessary equipment to conduct an enema. Even a simple enema without MMS can be beneficial. Regular bowel cleansing is considered a matter of course in Indian culture. It is important to find a balance here. Taking numerous enemas every day for weeks and months can put the bowels out of sync. My general advice would be to obtain the necessary equipment and try it out slowly to see how things go. Then, when you really need it, or if you want to administer it to a child, you have everything ready and you know what to do and what the difficulties are. Because of the MMS, the irrigator should not be made of metal or enamel – use a plastic one.

8.5 MMS FOOT BATHS

Double the quantity of activator

An MMS foot bath is an excellent way of detoxifying the body if oral administration is proving problematic.

You need a clean foot bath without trace of soap or other residues, as is the case with the full bath. First, as a starting dose, prepare ten drops of MMS with double the quantity of activator. You use twice the amount of activator so that much chlorine dioxide is released quickly, which means that you don't need to spend two hours bathing your feet.

Take ten drops of MMS and 20 drops of 3–5% hydrochloric acid or 50% tartaric acid and wait 40–60 seconds. Or if you are using citric acid as an activator, take 10 drops of MMS and 20 drops of 50% citric acid and wait 40–60 seconds. If no 1:1 activator is available you should still double the quantity of activator. For example when using 10% citric acid, take 100 drops (instead of the usual 50) to activate and then wait for 3 minutes. When the MMS is activated, top up the glass with water and put it in the foot bath you have prepared. Bathe your feet in it for at least 30 minutes. The quantity of water is not a decisive factor in the process. Take care to ensure that the temperature of the water is comfortable. If you easily tolerate ten drops, increase to 15 drops the next time, then 20 drops. After a number of baths with 20 drops, it may even be advisable to increase to 30, 40, 50 or 60 drops, depending on your individual case. Test it for yourself to see how much is good for you as an individual. Foot baths can be taken a number of times a day, if desired.

8.6 MMS eye drops

Jim Humble recommends the following procedure if you want to prepare MMS eye drops to treat eye diseases or inflammation.

Take two drops of MMS and activate them with a reduced quantity of acid. When the activation period has passed, add 200ml of water. Then pour the diluted MMS solution into a small, brown glass bottle, for example 20, 30, or 50ml with a pipette lid. Draw the solution into the pipette and drip one to two drops into the affected eye, or into both eyes. Then keep your eyes closed for about five minutes. It is not necessary to rinse out the eyes.

Keep in mind that chlorine dioxide bleaches. Keep a paper handkerchief at the ready to prevent the chlorine dioxide from dripping from your eyes and onto your clothes. If you are self-administering the eye drops it is easiest to do so in the bathroom, where you can administer the drops partially dressed, leaning the head back. If you have someone to help you it is easiest to do it lying down. If you use a bed or a sofa you could place a white towel under your head and keep a handkerchief at the ready. This will prevent your upholstery from becoming stained if a drop goes astray. In my opinion it is best to treat chronic eye conditions at least twice a day, once in the morning and once in the evening. With acute eye diseases you can administer the eye drops as often as you think necessary, although I would advise against using it more than twelve times in one day. As when administering MMS in any other way, you assume full responsibility when using MMS as an eye drop. The use of MMS as an eye drop, as well as the size and frequency of doses, should be adjusted to your individual level of sensitivity; decide what you consider to be suitable for you.

If you are not sure whether or not MMS eye drops are helping you, it is advisable to consult an eye specialist. I recommend making yourself familiar with the basic principles of MMS use (see chapters 6 and 7) before using MMS eye drops.

One more suggestion: eye drops of any kind feel strange the first time you use them. I therefore recommend you use a few drops of an isotonic saline solution or an eye-rinse solution before using the MMS eye drop, so that you become used to the feeling of using eye drops, and to the practical difficulties that arise, such as drops running astray. It is easier than it sounds, and with a little practise using MMS eye drops is quite easy.

If you intend to use the MMS eye drops multiple times a day, put the MMS eye drop solution in a brown glass pipette bottle and store it in a cool, dark place with the lid closed. When stored in this manner the solution can be used without significant loss of potency for a week. If it is not stored in a refrigerator you can still use it for one to two days; after that it is better to throw it away and prepare a new solution. You can buy brown glass pipette bottles in pharmacies. Sizes ranging from 10 to 50ml are suitable for preparing eye drops. The less 'empty' space left in the bottle, the more chlorine dioxide stays in the water solution; the warmer it is, the more chlorine dioxide takes a gaseous form and escapes when you open the bottle.

8.7 MMS IN INTRAVENOUS INFUSIONS

Infusions should not be carried out by laypersons, only by qualified professionals such as doctors, alternative practitioners and suitably trained nurses, carers and medical assistants.

The advantage of infusions is that they bypass the gastrointestinal tract and the portal venous system, thus allowing relatively large quantities of chlorine dioxide to be administered. In addition, infusions make it possible to administer precise dosages, minimising the danger of error in application. Infusions enable those who cannot tolerate MMS as a drink or who have gastrointestinal problems, as well as multimorbid or seriously ill patients, to receive a highly effective treatment.

Highly effective treatment

In my opinion, the administration of MMS by infusion should be restricted to those mentioned above. Other users are better advised to stick to oral administration and baths, if they tolerate these well. Taking MMS spread over the course of the day in accordance with the new standard protocol (see page 106) has proven successful even against serious illnesses. If it is not possible to take MMS orally for whatever reason, intravenous infusion is a good alternative.

Jim Humble and various other people have tested activated MMS intravenously. However, it became apparent that MMS activated with lemon juice damages the veins. Jim Humble therefore began recommending using unactivated MMS for intravenous applications, and then only under specialist supervision, that is, with a doctor or alternative practitioner present. This procedure was better tolerated by the veins but often led to Herxheimer reactions, presumably because of impurities in the substance infused. I therefore regard this method as obsolete and advise against it.

The alternative practitioner Dr Hartmut Fischer has experimented with infusions on himself and on his students and has developed a procedure which he has also successfully used on patients – **this has never caused Herxheimer reactions.**

Preparing MMS for infusions is a **completely different procedure** to that used when preparing it for oral administration. Firstly, the liquids used intravenously may not contain any pyrogens (impurities that cause fever). Secondly, the solution's pH-value must be compatible with that of the blood, meaning that it is vital that there is no excess activator. This is not an issue when taking MMS orally.

Because MMS infusions offer increased application possibilities and excellent efficacy, it is a very valuable treatment and the additional effort is worth it in cases of serious illnesses. To this end, Dr Fischer (see index of therapists) uses sterile nano-filters as used in biochemical laboratories. They have a Luer adapter and therefore fit onto current syringes. In this way the MMS is filtered as it is drawn up. The MMS is activated using

Dr Fischer

Pharmaceu- pharmaceutical grade acid. A stoichiometric calculator must be used to
tical grade determine the exact quantity of the chosen activator to correspond to
acid the desired number of drops of MMS. Activation takes place directly in
the syringe by drawing in the set quantity of acid, which is also filtered
through the sterilised nano-filter. Alternatively, the MMS can be activated in a sterilised sample bottle as used for liquid chromatography.
The solution is then prediluted with sterile water and drawn back up
into the syringe. MMS prepared in this way can then, using a new sterile
cannula, be added to the infusion bottle through the septum. The prepared infusions must be kept in a dark place until they are used.

Training Medical professionals, doctors and alternative practitioners interested in attending a training course can contact Dr Hartmut Fischer.

Dioxychlor™ A chlorine dioxide solution for infusions is produced in the USA under the name 'Dioxychlor'. Every now and again you come across doctors and clinics that work with it. To find up-to-date information, use internet search engines to look for terms such as 'Dioxychlor infusions' or 'MMS infusions'. Dioxychlor™ was developed and optimised by scientists at the Bradford Research Institute in close collaboration with Stanford University, the National Cancer Institute and the Mayo Clinic. With more than 50,000 infusions carried out across the globe, it has proved its efficacy against various illnesses.

This procedure was used at the Swiss Seegarten Clinic until a few years ago. You can still find interesting information on their website www.seegartenklinik.ch if you search under 'Dioxychlor'.

Summary of Through the formation of oxygen atoms (O_1), chlorine dioxide destroys
the website viruses, bacteria and fungi; in the case of the poliovirus, for example, at a concentration of less than 1ppm (parts per million: the unit of concentration that describes the quantity of an active / harmful agent in 1 million parts). Since chlorine dioxide destroys the guanine nucleotide bases of the RNA and DNA that is released, the formation of new generations of pathogens is halted. (Author's note: resistant strains cannot develop as a result.) However, chlorine dioxide is not cytotoxic. Various viral, bacterial, and fungal infections are listed as indications, as well as the side effects of antibiotic treatment; there are no known contraindications.
(Source: www.seegartenklinik.ch/?search=dioxychlor#)

It is likely that every high-purity chlorine dioxide solution is suitable for infusions. In future, it would be desirable to have studies carried out on this at various hospitals and clinics.

8.8 Nasal inhalation of MMS

I do not recommend this method because it is not without risk. Jim Humble does not recommend it either. One inhalation too many, or too deep, can be harmful.

Pure chlorine dioxide gas is far more reactive than chlorine dioxide solution and it behaves very differently. The reason for this is that the red blood cells do not distinguish between oxygen and chlorine dioxide. When inhaling, you would take in too much chlorine dioxide gas too quickly, which could pose a danger of suffocation. That cannot happen when drinking the liquid at the recommended dose. On the contrary, the body takes advantage of the fact that the red blood cells transport the chlorine dioxide to the seat of the disease. As with everything, the dose is the difference between being a cure or a poison.

Careful! Chlorine dioxide gas is poisonous.

That is why **chlorine dioxide gas is classed as being highly poisonous**, while chlorine dioxide solutions containing up to 2g/l ClO_2 are easy to handle and are stable for a number of days. However, that does not mean that such doses of chlorine dioxide solutions should be used internally. The statement refers to storage life and industrial use. Since both Jim Humble and I have experimented with this, we want to share our experiences. You can then decide for yourself whether or not you want to undertake experiments with chlorine dioxide gas on your own responsibility. We advise against it.

Jim Humble clears his respiratory passages before breakfast every day. He activates two drops of MMS with ten drops of 10% citric acid. He does not add water. As soon as the smell of chlorine dioxide is perceptible, he places the glass under his nose and inhales the chlorine dioxide gas slowly. He takes the gas into the nose and sinuses four times. He then takes in at least four slow breaths of fresh air without chlorine dioxide. Then he breathes normally again. He emphasises that only two drops should be activated – no more.

DEEP INHALATIONS CAN HARM THE LUNGS.

If you do want to try it, breathe in slowly and only inhale the chlorine dioxide into the nose, not deep into the lungs.

This method temporarily reduces the oxygen available in the body because chlorine dioxide is transported in the red blood cells as if it were oxygen. **MMS inhalations should, therefore, not be used if you have angina pectoris, are short of breath, or if you receive additional oxygen as part of your treatment.** Take care too if you suffer from asthma.

You should avoid inhaling MMS if you have taken more than 10 drops of MMS internally (with water) within the last two hours. If you do not suffer from the problems mentioned above, you could try inhaling MMS. **The following should always be observed:**

Synopsis **Only activate two drops, take four slow, shallow breaths into the nose and the sinuses. Do not inhale more than four times. Then take four slow breaths of fresh air so that your body is supplied with enough oxygen.**

If you experience irritation or light-headedness, you should of course stop. Those with sensitive eyes should keep their eyes closed so that the conjunctiva does not become irritated. If you follow these instructions you should be able to inhale chlorine dioxide gas without much risk. However, it is difficult to say exactly because we are all individuals and no large study has ever been carried out.

This application helps with chronic and acute respiratory infections and with inflammation of the neck, throat, and vocal chords. The chlorine dioxide reaches the affected areas and oxidises the pathogens much more quickly than it can when taken orally. In cases of illness, our experiences indicate that a good approach is to repeat the procedure every one to two hours. Acute infections usually respond very quickly. Consider this carefully: if you inhale chlorine dioxide gas into the nose, you do so at your own risk and on your own responsibility. Be very careful.

Stick to two drops: this will almost certainly be enough to have a curative effect. Any more could be dangerous.
The 2-drop mixture should not be swallowed.
It burns if no water is added.

After his morning inhalations, Jim Humble uses the two activated drops to brush his teeth.

If you suffer from an illness, once you have inhaled the MMS you could add a minimum of 180ml of water to the two drops after the activation period and drink it. Keep in mind your nausea threshold. Inhaling chlorine dioxide gas will quickly cause a large amount of chlorine dioxide to circulate in the body and can, under certain circumstances, lead to nausea. If that is the case, it is better not to take anything orally in addition: simply throw away the two activated drops if you don't need them to brush your teeth with. When the nausea has abated try again using just one drop.

8.9 Cleansing spaces with MMS

Activated MMS should **not** be put in humidifiers. It is odourless when it is in a water solution so will not bother you in that regard but constantly inhaling chlorine dioxide for long periods of time, even in small quantities, can lead to a lack of oxygen in the body and subsequently to dangerous situations. If you want to remove mould and fungi from the air in a room, you should not remain there for long periods. Pets and birds should also be taken out of the room before you place the bowl with activated MMS in it in a room. Close all doors and windows. To cleanse a room, simply place a cup or bowl (of glass, porcelain or plastic, not metal) containing 10 to 20 drops of activated MMS (without adding water) in the centre of a room, close all doors and windows, and leave the room for an hour to allow the chlorine dioxide gas to do its work. If you have a ventilator, put it on to distribute the chlorine dioxide gas evenly around the room.

Caution: lack of oxygen

Chlorine dioxide gas does not leave any unpleasant odours in curtains, drapery or upholstery. When the gas has evaporated, the odour will also disappear. Throw the activated MMS mixture away when you return to the room and rinse out the container. Then ventilate the room thoroughly.

8.10 Using MMS in a gas bag

This application method was specially developed to treat Morgellons disease, a parasitic disease in which worms crawl out of the skin, causing areas of the skin to become inflamed. Jim Humble developed this additional procedure because Morgellons patients experienced no relief from the existing MMS application methods.

You will need You will need two large bin bags, a container that has enough space in it for a large desert bowl, but small enough that you can place it at the bottom of the bin bag with room enough for your feet at its sides. The bin bags need to be big enough for you to be able to climb into them.

Cut open the bottom of the second bin bag and tape the two bin bags together with a strongly adhesive, gas-proof tape. The extended bin bags should now be big enough for any adult to be able to stand in it with the top of the bag sealed around the neck. You will certainly need a second person to help you and to keep the bag sealed around your neck because your arms should be in the bag. It is best to try this out in advance. You will then need an open bowl with activated MMS. Start with four drops and, if you tolerate it well, increase slowly to 20 drops. The open bowl with activated MMS releases chlorine dioxide in gas form. Because the gas cannot escape from the bag its effect on the skin is relatively concentrated and it can quickly reach the parasites in deeper layers via the channels that the parasites themselves have tunnelled. The gas bag should be kept sealed around the neck for about 15 minutes.

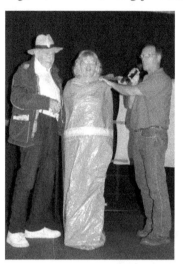

Warning: danger of suffocation **The bag should never be placed over the head. The nose and mouth must always be free to breathe normally, that is, the head must not be covered. Otherwise there is a danger of suffocation.**

It is best to stand naked in the gas bag. It makes it easier and quicker for the chlorine dioxide to reach the skin, with the added advantage that your clothes will not be bleached. If you want to use MMS in a gas bag, follow the instructions below.

Instructions Activate four drops of MMS in an open bowl. Place the bowl in a container. Climb, with help, into the extended bin bag. When the activation time is over, place the container with the bowl at the bottom of the gas sack and stand over it or at its side. If that is not possible, you can also hold the container with bowl in your hands. It is important that the bowl does not topple over. The person helping you should now seal the top of the bag as tightly as possible around your neck so that as little gas as possible escapes. The person helping you should take care not to press on your larynx or other sensitive parts of the throat. It works best if you seal the bag directly beneath the lower jaw and chin, especially with people who cannot tolerate constriction around the neck. This way you will not be pressing on the neck at all.

The gas sack can be used a number of times a day, depending on individual tolerance and level of urgency. If possible, increase the dose slowly from four to 20 drops. In Morgellons cases, it will be necessary to apply the treatment over an extended period of time. Some patients experienced good results after using the gas bag. For all other problems that you wish to treat with MMS, oral and external use is more efficient.

8.11 Disinfecting water

One drop of activated MMS or one to two drops of 0.29% chlorine dioxide solution (CDS) per litre is enough to disinfect water, depending on the degree of contamination. You should wait for up to 30 minutes after applying the solution so that the microbes are eliminated. Consume the water within two days, or add another drop of activated MMS or one to two drops of 0.29% chlorine dioxide solution per litre once again. *1 drop per litre of water*

You can find MMS tablets on the internet, also known as MMS effervescent tablets. Their advantage is that they are easier to transport on flights and, in addition to purifying water, can be used internally on your own responsibility. *Tablets*

MMS tablets or MMS effervescent tablets can be split. For example, a quarter 100ppm-strength tablet dissolved in a litre of water yields Jim Humble's recommended daily dose (+/- 24ppm) of chlorine dioxide per litre of water. You can also prepare smaller doses for yourself based on these figures.

For example, you could drink one-third of this litre (containing one-quarter of a tablet) one day, thereby taking the equivalent of eight drops of activated MMS. In this way you can use water purification tablets according to your needs to produce activated MMS of various strengths. Use the MMS to purify the air in your home, in sick rooms, storage cupboards or animal sheds, as a deodorant, as a preservative etc.

One disadvantage is that the tablets currently available on the market lose potency over time, despite being sealed in foil. Tests have shown that tablets that originally contained 100ppm chlorine dioxide only contained 42ppm after being stored for about three months. So further research is needed here.

8 • *More ways of administering MMS*

Air travel

If you want to buy MMS tablets to take on journeys when travelling by air, I would advise you to ask internet retailers who supply MMS in liquid form whether they also sell tablets, or search for MMS tablets and ask whether reliable tests have been done regarding how long they remain effective. If no reliable information is available regarding the quantities of chlorine dioxide produced, it is very difficult to administer precise doses. In that case I would recommend taking a small amount of MMS, 10ml for example, with you on your journey and activate it with fresh lemon juice.

Dual-component powder

Alternatively, you have the option of working with a powder. You can buy the 'Good for Life' water purifier in a PE bottle as a preprepared dose for 100ml of water. When required, you then only need to fill up the bottle with warm water and wait for the reaction time of four hours to pass. However, there are issues regarding loss of efficacy, depending on time and temperature ratios. This is because the powder in the bottle forms chlorine dioxide gas before the addition of water. This gas escapes when you open the bottle, if not before. The chlorine dioxide solution produced with this method, as with all other chlorine dioxide solutions, should be sealed and stored in a cool, dark place. In my opinion it should also be used within a few weeks. But be aware that this chlorine dioxide solution contains at least about 20 times less chlorine dioxide than normal MMS.

8.12 Disinfecting food

If you suspect that E. coli or other pathogens are being spread in food, you can disinfect your food using MMS.

Use the following procedure.

5 drops in 1 litre of water

Activate 5 drops of MMS in a container made of glass, plastic or ceramic and add a litre of water once the activation time has passed. If you need more water, use correspondingly greater quantities of MMS (e.g. ten drops of MMS in two litres of water, 15 drops of MMS in three litres of water etc.). Then place the food you want to disinfect in the MMS water, completely covering the food with water. Depending on the weight of the food, you may have to weigh it down with a suitable object so that parts that float upwards are adequately submerged. Take the food out of the water after ten minutes and rinse thoroughly with water. You can then consume it.

Food disinfected using MMS in this way tastes good. A few small 'wrinkles' sometimes appear on the outer skin of tomatoes, apples and cucumbers. I have not noticed any visible changes to carrots, lettuce or cabbage. Jim Humble claims that there is no difference in taste between food washed with MMS and that washed with normal tap water. I have tested this by washing tomatoes, carrots, cucumbers, apples, lettuce and cabbage with MMS water and have found that some of the taste is lost, but the difference is subtle. There is absolutely no chlorine taste. All the food tasted great, both raw and cooked, leading me to suspect that people who do not regularly eat organic foods would not have noticed any difference.

I therefore consider this procedure for disinfecting food with MMS to be a simple, safe and cheap alternative to complete abstinence from food at times when you are unsure whether food is contaminated or not.

Moreover, sodium chlorite has been approved and recognised as being completely safe for use as a food disinfectant by the FDA in the USA, where it is in standard use.

8.13 CHLORINE DIOXIDE SOLUTION (CDS)

It has by now become possible to produce a solution which contains pure chlorine dioxide dissolved in water.

That has many advantages:
1. You only need one bottle.
2. The activation process in no longer necessary and, as a result, the potential for excess acid is eliminated; nausea almost never occurs.
3. There is less of an odour problem.
4. It tastes considerably better.
5. It is purer, containing only water and chlorine dioxide.
6. When diluted appropriately, it is probably much better than MMS for intravenous use.
7. It can also be used intramuscularly on animals.

This solution was developed by Andreas Kalcker, a biophysicist, filmmaker and author, when he was asked by a calf breeder for a special solution. The calf breeder faced a problem: he needed a number of medicines for his calves – a situation which was financially untenable. However, MMS could not be administered because of the resulting stomach problems.

Distillation process Chlorine dioxide is produced in a distillation process of two components in the conventional manner as with MMS; the gas produced is bound in cool water. Using this process, it is possible to produce a 0.29% pure chlorine dioxide solution. Since using the wrong tube materials can cause an explosion, I cannot recommend that laypersons carry out this procedure. Those interested can learn the process in courses given by Jim Humble.

A pure chlorine dioxide solution should not be confused with the chlorine dioxide solution produced from a two-component powder such as 'Good for Life'. That is also a chlorine dioxide solution but the chlorine dioxide has not been produced through a distillation process, meaning that other substances are also present.

Application

Cool before use Caution! Before opening the chlorine dioxide solution for the first time, you must put the bottle in the refrigerator for a few hours to cool it. This causes the chlorine dioxide to bind more firmly with the water, reducing the amount that can escape. This should also be done if the bottle of chlorine dioxide has, for whatever reason, become warm again. It is important to close the bottle immediately after use and to put it back in the refrigerator. The chlorine dioxide solution loses its efficacy mainly when the bottle is opened, especially when the bottle has been exposed to light or heat beforehand.

No activation Unlike MMS, the chlorine dioxide solution does not need to be activated. You only need to count the required number of drops and add water – no juice.

Undiluted CDS can be applied externally Externally, CDS can be applied undiluted to the skin and the lips. If it burns, rinse it away.

Dose

The dose recommendations given here refer to the chlorine dioxide solution available today, and have been compiled based on my own experience and the experience of other users. They offer a point of orientation and are not to be regarded as a medical prescription by any means. In individual circumstances, it may be advisable to take much higher doses.

It is for you to decide whether you want to take chlorine dioxide solution on your own responsibility, and how much of it you want to take.

With the aid of a photometer we have measured the chlorine dioxide content of 0.29% chlorine dioxide solutions supplied by four different suppliers. In each case, we put six drops in a glass with 250ml of water. We measured values ranging from 0.17mg chlorine dioxide/litre to 5.76mg chlorine dioxide/litre. The same quantity of MMS activated in the standard 1:1 ratio (albeit for only 20 seconds) with tartaric acid in 250ml of water yielded 9.52mg of chlorine dioxide.

Large variation in values

As you can see, the difference in strength is enormous. Presumably other chlorine dioxide solutions will be available soon. Since we do not know how strong the chlorine dioxide solution obtained from them is, we can only recommend starting on a low dose and increasing slowly, as when taking MMS, for example 2 drops, then 5 drops, then 8 drops, and so forth until you can feel it having a positive effect. Never take more than you can tolerate comfortably. Depending on the strength of the solution, you may want to take 30, 40, 50, 60 drops or more per dose, to obtain a positive effect. The situation is at an experimental stage in terms of dosage.

With malaria (and indeed with any illness if you are of the opinion that the chlorine dioxide solution is not strong enough), it is advisable to revert to using the normal MMS, since experience shows that taking 15 drops of activated MMS once or twice is certainly enough to cure malaria.

Loss of efficacy / storage

According to the manufacturers' instructions, the chlorine dioxide solutions currently available will keep for a maximum of six months when stored in a cool, dark place (below 11°C, ideally in the refrigerator). However, the solution is always weakening – you will know from the way the yellow colour fades over time, especially if exposed to light, air and heat, which is inevitable every time you take it out of the refrigerator. That makes it difficult to determine what constitutes a suitable dose with regard to individual tolerance, and the effective number of drops. I can therefore only recommend the chlorine dioxide solutions currently available if you intend to use the product within a few weeks. Despite these uncertainties, many users are ardent advocates of chlorine dioxide solution.

Chlorine dioxide solution should, of course, be stored out of the reach of children.

Observe the following guidelines to minimise any loss of efficacy.
1. Before opening the bottle for the first time, place it in the refrigerator and cool to a temperature of about 11 °C.
2. Close the bottle again directly after use and put it back in the refrigerator.
3. When transporting, always protect from light and heat, and/or, after transporting, leave to cool to about 11 °C in the refrigerator before use.

What to consider when buying CDS

You should ask two questions when buying a chlorine dioxide solution.
1. Is it really a pure, distilled chlorine dioxide solution dissolved in water and not a powder or a sodium chlorite solution?
2. Have any studies been carried out on the solution's chlorine dioxide content, and on how the strength of the solution changes over time, from which conclusions can be drawn regarding how long the potency of the solution remains constant?

If in doubt, the colour of the solution will tell you whether or not it contains chlorine dioxide. If it is yellowish, then there is chlorine dioxide present. If it is colourless, then the chlorine dioxide has escaped or was never present.

Unfortunately, the difference in colour between a 0.3% solution and a 0.03% solution is not particularly great, which means that you cannot accurately judge the quantitative strength based solely on colour. The colour only tells you whether or not there is any chlorine dioxide present, and can only roughly estimate its quantity.

Violet glass bottles When buying bottles look for good-quality bottles. It seems that storing chlorine dioxide in violet glass bottles is best in terms of preserving potency.

Experiences

The following findings, summarised in short points, draw on my own personal experience or the experience of colleagues who have carried out experiments on themselves.
- Everyone who has previously taken MMS says that pure chlorine dioxide solution tastes better than MMS, and that it was effective, although in some cases only after big increases in doses.

Chlorine dioxide solution (CDS)

- Regarding one of the chlorine dioxide solutions tested, 10–40 drops had to be used a number of times a day to have any effect.
- The same solution was less effective than MMS at a dosage of 4:1 in proportion to MMS; some users therefore preferred to use MMS, while other users had good results despite only using double or four times the number of drops.
- Some colleagues were so enthusiastic about the taste and tolerability of the pure chlorine dioxide solution that they now prefer to use chlorine dioxide solution since they were also satisfied with its efficacy.
- Results were quickly achieved with the following illnesses: acholia, arthritis, bronchitis, corneous / broken / raw skin, herpes labialis, nail fungus, otitis, rhinitis, senile warts, sinusitis, suppurative tonsillitis. No experience report is yet available regarding the most serious illnesses.

I therefore recommend that those who wish to try out chlorine dioxide solution use the established dosage recommendation for MMS as a point of orientation when using chlorine dioxide solution. Start conservatively with 2–5 drops (instead of between one-half of a drop and one drop of MMS) before increasing to 8 drops, then to 10 drops, and if necessary even higher, so that you are then, as with the new standard protocol, taking the desired number of drops of chlorine dioxide solution per hour (instead of 3 drops of MMS per hour).

If, however, the colour of the solution has paled after some time, you can no longer rely on this dosage pattern. You could then increase the dose further based on effect or, ideally, buy a new bottle.

If you prefer taking a different dose you can certainly do so, but I would advise you to take care when increasing the dose and to test how much you can tolerate. At this present time the highest single dose taken without adverse reactions that is known to me, is 70 drops; this does not, of course, mean that that would be possible for everyone. As our tests have shown, the chlorine dioxide solution labelled 0.3% did not contain anywhere near 0.3% chlorine dioxide. Some animals can tolerate significantly higher doses of this weaker chlorine dioxide solution; one 65kg dog, for example, was cured with multiple doses of 200 drops daily. However, if you have a chlorine dioxide solution with a high chlorine dioxide content this dose could prove to be too high.

Inaccurate information

Summary

Opinion is divided on chlorine dioxide solution produced by distillation. Some love it because of its simplicity (no activation and therefore no acid necessary), good tolerability, and a pleasant taste. Others dislike it, mainly because of the limited time the solution remains reliably effective, and because of the lower levels of potency. But the number of advocates of chlorine dioxide solution (CDS) is growing due to the positive results experienced from its use.

8.14 GEFEU SOLUTION

Improvement in taste This is an alternative to standard MMS activation which also increases the yield of chlorine dioxide and improves the taste.

Producing a chlorine dioxide solution from MMS and an activator using a method developed by Gerhard Feustle, the so-called 'Gefeu solution', is less time-consuming than producing distilled chlorine dioxide solution. This is, however, not a pure chlorine dioxide solution since it is not produced through distillation. The Gefeu method offers three advantages over Jim Humble's activation process, allowing you to save time and money.

1. You only need about five minutes to carry out the activation once, and then you will have a large quantity of ready-to-use chlorine dioxide solution with a level of potency that will remain stable for at least three to four weeks (if stored in a closed container in a cool, dark place).
2. There is no excess of acid to cause problems.
3. You obtain about three times the amount of chlorine dioxide from one bottle of MMS because Jim Humble's activation method allows much of the chlorine dioxide produced to escape into the air in the form of gas. The Gefeu method has the advantage that when activated, the chlorine dioxide gas produced is instantly bound to the water and is available in the dose you take.

You will find interesting explanations and detailed instructions (in German) on how to produce chlorine dioxide solution using the Gefeu method on the MMS self-help forum under the title 'Anwendungsfälle – Neues aus Gefeus Chlordioxidlabor' (www.mms-selbsthilfe.de/showthread. php?1437-Neues-aus-gefeu-s-Chlordioxid-Labor). Below is a slightly modified summary of the Gefeu method.

Gefeu solution

You will need one 100ml dark glass bottle, two 20ml dark glass bottles with a dripper or pipette lid, a 10ml syringe, a cannula (needle) that is at least 3.5cm long and as thick as possible, some cold water, a cooled bottle of MMS and cooled activator.

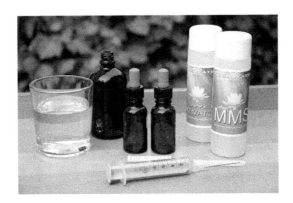

1. In a syringe, draw up 40ml of water (4 x 10ml) from a clean glass of water and place in a 100ml dark glass bottle. Place the bottle in the refrigerator.
2. Draw up (using the same disposable syringe) exactly 2ml sodium chlorite solution; wipe the needle with a clean paper towel.
3. Directly afterwards, draw up exactly 1ml of 50% tartaric acid or 3-5% hydrochloric acid into the same syringe.
4. During the activation time, place the needle of the syringe in the cooled glass bottle (hold the bottle at a slight angle, almost flat). The chlorine dioxide gas that comes out of the syringe is instantly bound by the water. Wait 40 to 60 seconds.
5. Now inject the entire mixture into the glass bottle – swirl briefly to mix.
6. Decant the content of the bottle into the two 20ml bottles, then close them with a dropper lid or a pipette lid. Label the bottles, indicating their content ('Gefeu solution') and date; store them in the refrigerator. If you leave the 40ml in the 100ml bottle, over the course of time chlorine dioxide will escape into the space within the bottle and will be lost when the bottle is opened; less is lost with smaller bottles.

Bear in mind that the 'Gefeu solution' is a chlorine dioxide concentrate. I strongly advise the following:

never drink it pure, and always mix the desired number of drops in a glass of water.

Summary of the possible ways of obtaining chlorine dioxide

Method	Advantages	Disadvantages	Dosage (Number of drops compared to 1 drop of activated MMS 1)
MMS 1 + activator 1:1	Simple method, most effective, tried and tested	Activation necessary, taste, smell, relatively low tolerance threshold	1
MMS 1 + reduced acid activation 1:0.5	Simple method, tried and tested, less excess acid, improved taste	Activation necessary, taste, smell, relatively low tolerance threshold	1
Gefeu solution	Increased chlorine dioxide yield, less excess acid, much improved taste	Activation necessary, c. 5 minutes preparation the first time, not a pure chlorine dioxide solution	7 (approx.) Can vary depending on different drop sizes and the preparation. Start with one drop and increase if you can tolerate it.
Slow activation based on the Fischer method	Pleasanter taste, easier to prepare than the Gefeu solution	Activation necessary, not immediately available – can only be taken after at least 4 hours, ideally after 8 to 12 hours, not a pure chlorine dioxide solution	1 (presumed same effectiveness due to post-activation in the body)
2-component powder, currently only available to retailers in large quantities (sodium chlorite and activator)	Long shelf life when unopened	Activation necessary, not immediately available – can only be taken after at least 4 hours, ideally after 8 to 12 hours, not a pure chlorine dioxide solution because it is not produced using a distillation process	At least 10

Method	Advantages	Disadvantages	Dosage (Number of drops compared to 1 drop of activated MMS 1)
'Good for Life' – water steriliser, 2-component powder mixed into one component	Simple method	Activation by adding water necessary, not immediately available – can only be taken after at least 4 hours, ideally after 8 to 12 hours, not a pure chlorine dioxide solution because it is not produced using a distillation process, soon loses effectiveness because both components are delivered together as a pre-mixed powder.	At least 10
MMS + activator 1:1 + sodium bicarbonate	Simple method, less excess acid, significantly improved taste, substances have a long shelf life without cool storage, more reliable dosage.	Activation necessary The chlorine dioxide content is drastically reduced when too much sodium bicarbonate is used	1
Chlorine dioxide solution (CDS) produced through distillation	No activation necessary, the simplest method, no excess acidity, pleasant taste, good tolerance threshold, purest variety available.	Sensitive to light and heat, must be stored in a cool place after opening, doses are only reliable for a few weeks, doses of about 2 to 10 times higher are required.	2 to 10 or more; big fluctuation depending on the manufacturer.

It is impossible to draw a direct comparison in terms of doses because there is a huge variation in the strength of the solutions produced when activating by using Jim Humble's procedure, dependent on the activator and activation time. As a general point of orientation, one drop of Gefeu solution is about seven times weaker than one drop of activated MMS. (But since you obtain 20 drops of Gefeu solution from one drop of MMS, you have effectively tripled the quantity of chlorine dioxide from one drop of MMS.) These figures refer to photometric measurements of chlorine dioxide values in a Gefeu solution prepared as I have just described, compared to the same quantity of MMS activated 1:1 with 50% tartaric acid.

Since you are aiming for the optimal number of drops for you as an individual, you can use any of Jim Humble's protocols for dosing as long as you always start with one drop, and pay attention to your tolerance threshold. If you keep the Gefeu solution well sealed in a refrigerator, it retains its full potency for at least three to four weeks. After that, it can still be used with good effect for another two months – increase the number of drops if necessary.

Advantages By using the Gefeu method, you substantially increase the yield of chlorine dioxide, and the taste is much more pleasant than that achieved by the standard activation process.

This method of DIY chlorine dioxide solution production is ideally suited to those who like to tinker and to experiment. Others are probably better served with a ready-to-use CDS, standard activation in accordance with Jim Humble's method (ideally with reduced acid), or slow activation based on the Fischer method, because of their simplicity.

8.15 MMS ENERGY GLOBULES

MMS energy globules are energetically imprinted pills, similar to homeopathic remedies. They are available in various strengths: 1 drop per hour, 3 drops per hour, 6 drops per hour, 6 drops per hour 6 times a day, and 8 drops per hour from 5 p.m. to 9 p.m. The following CDS energy globule varieties are also available: 1 drop CDS per hour, 4 drops per hour, and 10 drops per hour. Biochemically speaking, they do not contain MMS. They are programmed to function energetically.

MMS energy globules are not meant to be taken internally but are carried on the body. It appears that they work through vibration transmission, although this has not yet been proven scientifically. You will find more information (in German) at:

www.informierteGlobuli.de

Conclusion

Having considered the respective advantages and disadvantages of each method, I recommend the following approaches, depending on your needs and priorities:
- MMS + reduced acid activation for all those who prefer fresh activation in order to have certainty regarding the strength, and who are not overly bothered by the acidity and the slightly acidic taste.
- CDS (chlorine dioxide solution) is best in terms of taste and tolerability. It is recommended for those who prefer the ease of use and those who cannot tolerate acid – but it must be taken at doses of about 2 to 10 times higher than standard MMS, it must be stored in a cool place, and used within 4 weeks of breaking the seal, up to a maximum of 6 months.
- Powder for journeys by air or if, for any other reason, solutions cannot be used.
- MMS energy globules for those who prefer treatment on an energetic level.

All the other methods of producing solutions containing chlorine dioxide described here also work well. Find out for yourself which is the most suitable for your needs.

MMS 2

MMS 2, like MMS, is only approved for use as a water steriliser, not as a medicine, therefore it cannot be prescribed and must be taken on your own responsibility.

In August 2009, Jim Humble announced on the internet that he had developed another mineral solution which he called MMS 2. For this, he takes calcium hypochlorite and activates it with water. This produces hypochlorous acid (HOCl), an acid that is produced by our immune systems to break down pathogens of all kinds and render them harmless. If, as Jim Humble reflected, the human body is unable to produce sufficient hypochlorous acid during an illness, it is to be expected that the administration of supplementary hypochlorous acid will significantly accelerate the healing process. On the basis of this hypothesis, Jim Humble first utilised hypochlorous acid in cases of prostate problems when a friend of his who had prostate cancer reported that the cancer had disappeared after using hypochlorous acid. According to Humble, good results were achieved for a variety of diseases. However, in comparison to MMS, the disadvantage of MMS 2 is that it not only kills pathogens but also the bacteria that support the body's normal physiological processes; that is, some of the 'good' bacteria can also be destroyed. Jim Humble specifically recommends using MMS 2 in addition to MMS in serious cases of illness where MMS alone is not enough to bring about a satisfactory state of health. It can be bought on the internet from some of the same suppliers who sell MMS.

Hypochlorous acid is used by the immune system

Jim Humble uses vegetable capsules size 0, filled with a 75% calcium hypochlorite powder from a local swimming pool equipment supplier. The concentration of calcium hypochlorite is usually between 45% and 85% and most swimming pool equipment suppliers sell calcium hypochlorite of about 75% by the sack. It is important that it really is calcium hypochlorite and not any other chlorine compound. This is because calcium hypochlorite becomes hypochlorous acid when it comes into contact with water. Swimming pool owners can thus use calcium hypo-

Available as a water steriliser

chlorite to sterilise pool water because it releases hypochlorous acid into the water. So water is the activator used to produce MMS 2.

If you decide to use it internally as a way of increasing the hypochlorous acid in your system, it is important, as with MMS, to increase the dose slowly.

If you are a very sensitive person I would even suggest you start with 30–50mg once a day, and only increase to 100mg once a day after ten days. I would advise you not to go any higher.

Also, if I were in your shoes, I would look for MMS 2 that fulfils the purity standards of the German Drinking Water Ordinance DIN EN 900 (or the equivalent in your country) just to be on the safe side.

Look after yourself; you know your own level of sensitivity. That is why you are the best judge of what your starting dose should be and how much your system can take. There is little sense in relying on others' experience if you know your body is much more sensitive.

Consider your individual level of sensitivity

Everyone can judge for themselves and, depending on their level of sensitivity, start at between 50 and 100mg – but only if you are ready to take full responsibility.

To find out how much calcium hypochlorite your body can tolerate, it is best to start with a capsule containing no more than 100mg. These are not available for sale at present. If you want to take calcium hypochlorite, you can do the following.

Buy capsules size 0 (approx. 400mg). Important: drink two glasses of water before taking it and drink another glass of water after taking it.

When taking it for the first time it is advisable to discard about three-quarters of the capsule's content. The capsule then contains about 100mg, which you swallow along with the capsule itself **(it is imperative that you first drink two glasses of water, then swallow the MMS 2 capsule, before drinking another glass of water)**. If you only want to take 50mg, halve this dose.

If you tolerate 100mg well, repeat that six times, that is, once a day, every day, for six days. Then, for the next two days only discard half the content. If that works well, take the whole capsule. The chances that you will tolerate it well are relatively high. If you experience adverse reactions when taking calcium hypochlorite even in small quantities you should not, on any account, increase the dose. You might be able to continue with a small dose (20–50mg) until taking calcium hypochlorite no longer causes any problems. After a while, it may be possible to increase a little more. Consider the benefits and the risks and decide for yourself.

9 • MMS 2

It is very important that you drink two glasses of water before taking a capsule, and that you drink another glass afterwards.

Activator   The water is necessary, firstly, as an activator and, secondly, the body needs more water to flush away the waste products. Imagine the water as a kind of garbage disposal system. What use would it be to renovate a house if the rubbish is not taken away? It can have severe consequences if the rubbish gets out of control and begins to pile up in all the rooms ... so be sure to drink enough water, and drink water between doses as well.

When you can tolerate one capsule well, on the following day you could try taking an additional capsule in the evening. When you have taken one capsule in the morning and one in the evening for two days (don't forget the water), you could increase to three or four capsules a day, as long as you continue to tolerate it well. Leave at least two hours between doses.

If you experience stomach aches, try drinking more water: it may be that the pain then disappears. If not, the only alternative is to stop taking the capsules, or to reduce the dose. It is, after all, better to proceed slowly and not to overtax your body. If in doubt, seek advice from your doctor or alternative practitioner.

Like MMS, MMS 2 is not an officially approved medication – it is a water steriliser. A doctor cannot prescribe it for you. But if you want to try it on your own responsibility, doctors can provide support and supervision, if they deem it to be appropriate.

I cannot advise you to take MMS 2, firstly because I don't know you, and secondly because I am not allowed to advise you to take something that is not officially intended for internal use.

However, since I know of many people who have used MMS 2 with good results, I certainly do not advise against using it. I provide information and leave it to you to take responsibility for whatever conclusions you draw. I do not accept any responsibility for any potential improvement or deterioration to your health that may result from taking MMS 2 on your own responsibility. MMS 2, like any other water steriliser – should be kept out of the reach of children. No interactions with other allopathic medicines have been observed so far.

Successful treatment of HIV   In Jim Humble's protocol for HIV, MMS 2 is taken in addition to MMS 1 (since MMS 2 has been available, some suppliers and users have started calling MMS 'MMS 1'): take three drops of activated MMS 1 eight times a day leaving at least an hour between doses; in addition, take one capsule of MMS 2 (capsule size 0) four times a day, half an hour after taking the MMS 1, leaving at least two hours between doses. Drink two glasses of water before taking the MMS 2 capsules, and another glass afterwards. Continue for three weeks and then have a blood test to determine the white blood cell count. In Jim Humble's experience, not all AIDS patients become healthy again when taking MMS on its own; but all AIDS patients tested by him who took both MMS **and** MMS 2 did.

In 2012 Jim Humble stated that he had used MMS 2 for five years to his full satisfaction.

Calcium hypochlorite must never be activated with water in the glass because the liquid produced, the hypochlorous acid, can burn the oesophagus. Activation must occur in the stomach: first drink two glasses of water, then swallow the MMS 2 capsule, followed by another glass of water.

DMSO AND MMS

Because MMS has been used very successfully in combination with DMSO, I wish to examine DMSO here in more detail. I will begin by explaining what DMSO is, and what users have reported after using it.

DMSO is an abbreviation of dimethyl sulfoxide ($CH_3 - SO - CH_3$), a colourless and odourless liquid that emanates a putrid smell after being stored for a long time. Because of its special ability to penetrate the skin it is often added to creams, gels, plasters and tinctures as a so-called drug delivery facilitator. Because DMSO itself has anti-inflammatory and painkilling properties, it is used in particular to treat rheumatic complaints and sports injuries. As with many substances, the dose is very important. At low concentrations it is safe for many people.

Dimethyl sulfoxide was first synthesised in 1866 by the Russian Alexander Saytzeff. Publication of his results followed in 1867 in a German chemistry journal. Since then, more than 11,000 scientific articles have been published worldwide regarding its medicinal application and more than 40,000 articles regarding its chemical properties. In the 1960s Dr Stanley Jacob from the Oregon Health Science University first identified the various therapeutic possibilities offered by DMSO.

He experimented with DMSO to optimise the preservation of transplanted organs and discovered that DMSO can penetrate the skin quickly and deeply without any damage to the skin. The following pharmacological properties have since been discovered:

Properties of DMSO
- Penetrates biological membranes
- Transports other molecules
- Influences the connective tissue
- Anti-inflammatory
- Nerve block (analgesic)
- Inhibition of bacterial growth (bacteriostatic)
- Diuretic

- Amplification or diminution of certain medicines
- Cholinesterase inhibitor
- General increase in resistance to infection
- Widening of blood vessels (vasodilation)
- Muscle relaxant
- Support of cell differentiation and cell function
- Inhibition of platelet agglutination (thrombocyte aggregation inhibitor)
- Protects biological tissue when exposed to radiation or frost
- Protects the tissue in cases of circulation problems

(Source: S. W. Jacob et al., Oregon Health Science University, Portland, Oregon)

DMSO's therapeutic spectrum is unusual. It has an anti-inflammatory and vasodilatory effect; it inhibits the growth of bacteria, fungi and viruses; it binds the free radicals that damage cells; it stimulates the immune system and promotes the healing of wounds; it even offers a certain level of protection against damage from x-rays and frost.

Read more about this in *DMSO: Nature's Healer* by Dr Morton Walker (New York: Avery, 1993).

The example cases described by Walker are particularly striking. For example, a 65-year-old woman went to a health centre in Auburndale, Florida, to receive treatment for a bursa inflammation in her right shoulder. Not only did the inflammation quickly abate but a phantom pain the patient had suffered ever since having her left leg amputated also disappeared. The head of the hospital, Dr Avery, who treated the patient, claims that the phantom pains have not returned in the ten years since. *Example cases* *Bursa inflammation* *Phantom pain*

The case of a woman with scleroderma is also striking. She had been suffering severe pains continuously for 19 years despite taking medication. A number of toes had been amputated. She noticed a significant palliation during the first week of DMSO treatment and after four months she had hardly any pains. She did not have to undergo any further amputations. *Scleroderma*

An article in *Der Spiegel* magazine (05/05/1965) describes the astounding swiftness with which DMSO takes effect on shoulder pains. Patients who were unable to dress and undress themselves because of pains resulting from bursa inflammations were free of pain, or almost free of pain, within 20 minutes of rubbing in DMSO. *Severe shoulder pains*
(Source: http://www.spiegel.de/spiegel/print/d-46272532.html)

Treating scar tissue with DMSO resulted in a regression of the scar tissue.

Regression of scar tissue
In 1967 J. F. Engle demonstrated that treating scar keloids with DMSO resulted in a move back towards 'normality', as shown by histological assessments. That was also what Dr Jörg Carls discovered, the man who, in cooperation with the Academy of Hand Rehabilitation, established the research project 'Topical application of DMSO on scars and illnesses from the spectrum of the Hannover Medical School / Annastift, Outpatients Surgical Clinic (AOZ)'. His conclusion: scar tissue regressed visibly and swelling abated significantly.
(Source: www.akademie-fuer-handrehabilitation.de/downloads/zwischenergebnissedesforschungsprojektesdmso.pdf, accessed May 2005)

DMSO was taken off the market by the American licensing authority, the FDA, in the 1960s because of animal testing. It later became apparent that damage to the lens of the eye, as had been observed in rabbits, dogs and pigs, did not occur in humans, even at high doses. Humans who were given doses 3 to 30 times the usual amount did not display significant side effects.

Side effects
Various skin reactions did occur, contrasting from individual to individual. In two of the 78 test persons there were elevated liver enzymes counts, 52% of the test subjects suffered from headaches, 42% became nauseous, 32% became drowsy, and 18% had burning eyes.

Those are indeed high percentages but it should be remembered that doses ranging from 3 to 30 times the normal amount were administered. Consider this: if you ate 3 to 30 times the normal amount of your favourite meal, headaches or nausea would tell you nothing regarding whether or not a normal portion is healthy for you.

Where physical symptoms did occur, they completely disappeared within three weeks. The study lasted three months and judged DMSO to be very safe. I have taken this information from Dr Jörg Carls' PDF document.
(Source: www.akademie-fuer-handrehabilitation.de/downloads/dmso.pdf)

That document contains detailed, specialist information regarding the toxicology of DMSO and treatment applications. For laypeople eager to know more, I would recommend reading Dr Morton Walker's book *DMSO: Nature's Healer* (Avery, 2000) and Dr Hartmut Fischer's book *The DMSO Handbook* (Daniel Peter Verlag, forthcoming 2015, ISBN 978-3-9815255-5-7).

If this has made you curious and you are keen to try DMSO for yourself, you can order it on the internet from a few suppliers who also sell MMS. When buying, look for **pharmaceutical quality** because DMSO is also used as an industrial solvent. Technical grade DMSO may contain considerable levels of impurities that penetrate the skin, potentially leading to unnecessary problems.

Test instructions

I urge you to bear in mind Jim Humble's experiences and first test to see whether you react allergically to DMSO. It can cause problems for people with poor liver function. So test first to see whether you can tolerate DMSO.

Jim Humble recommends the following procedure:
1. Wash your arm thoroughly.
2. When it is dry, put a drop of DMSO on a small patch of your arm and rub in the DMSO.
3. Leave for 15 minutes to be absorbed.
4. Wait a few hours.

If you do not experience liver pains or skin reactions after doing this, there is a 99% chance that you can tolerate DMSO.

If you want to be 100% certain, wait another 24 hours. If DMSO has caused a reaction do not use it.

Instructions

If you are able to tolerate DMSO, proceed as follows.
1. Activate MMS, for example ten drops MMS with ten drops of 3–5% hydrochloric acid or 50% tartaric acid.
2. Observe the activation time exactly. When using the above 1:1 activators wait 40–60 seconds and then add 1–2 teaspoons of water.
3. Immediately after the activation time has passed, add a teaspoon of DMSO, swirl the mixture and wait a maximum of 15 seconds.
4. Rub the mixture into the skin **within 15 seconds at the most**. Choose a large area on the extremities of your body to do this. Do it quickly: the mixture is continuously losing potency, a delay of just three minutes is too long. Jim Humble now recommends first spraying MMS onto the skin and rubbing in the DMSO on the same area afterwards. That way no valuable seconds are lost.

5. You can rub it in with your bare hands. If you feel it burning, dilute the mixture with more water. Rub in a teaspoon of water directly onto the area that burns. Use as many teaspoons of water as is needed to stop the burning. If the skin is a little irritated, soothe it with olive oil, aloe vera juice, or whatever helps your skin. It is a good idea to use a different area of skin each time you apply MMS and DMSO to the skin.
6. Do this every two hours on the first day and every hour on the second and third day. Take a break for four days. Then start again from the beginning.

During this time you should continue to take MMS orally within your individual tolerance threshold.

According to Jim Humble, adding DMSO to activated MMS causes up to five times as much MMS to be transported into deeper tissue layers in comparison to application without DMSO. **But this is only an advantage if you are able to tolerate it. Proceed carefully and prudently.**

That is also the advice when taking DMSO internally. In cases of severe illnesses such as strokes, Jim Humble recommends taking a level teaspoon of DMSO together with at least an equal amount of juice internally every quarter of an hour to an hour, and continuing to take the MMS doses. But in this case, the MMS should not be mixed with the DMSO. You can take one after the other. It is a matter of fully exploiting the time the DMSO is effective.

Only take DMSO internally after previously testing for tolerability.

Taking DMSO and MMS orally

If you are able to tolerate DMSO well, you can also take it internally to intensify the effect of MMS without problems.

The following procedure has proved useful and is called 'Protocol 1000+' by Jim Humble.
1. Activate between one and three drops of MMS and wait for the activation time to pass (this varies depending on the activator used).
2. Add at least 100ml of water, and tea or juice according to taste.
3. Then add between one and three drops of DMSO (one drop DMSO for each drop of MMS).

Have you passed the tolerability test? If so, you can drink MMS / DMSO on your own responsibility. Because DMSO has a strong antioxidant effect, it can reduce the oxidative power of chlorine dioxide if you leave the mixture for longer than five minutes.

If you are interested in reading more about the possible applications of DMSO, I recommend *The DMSO Handbook* by Dr Hartmut P. A. Fischer (Daniel Peter Verlag, forthcoming 2015, ISBN 978-3-9815255-5-7). It offers an excellent overview of everything you need to know about DMSO, including interesting example cases. *Reading suggestion*

11

Safety instructions for the use of
MMS, ClO₂, CDS, MMS 2 and DMSO

MMS, MMS 2 and DMSO are powerful substances – that is why they can be used to eliminate pathogens. As with any substance that is very effective, too much of it can be harmful. That is true even for sunshine and rain and it would never occur to us to say that sunshine or rain are generally dangerous.

It is the dosage that creates the poison. That has been known since time immemorial.

Pharmacological research uses laboratory animals, usually rats, to determine a substance's so-called LD value in order to classify its level of poisonousness. The LD_{50} value states what dose of a substance is lethal in 50% of cases. All the values in this example, with the exception of Lariam, refer to rats.

LD_{50} values

MMS (sodium chlorite) has an LD_{50} value of 250 to 500mg/kg of body weight.
ClO₂ (chlorine dioxide) has an LD_{50} value of 292mg/kg of body weight.
MMS 2 (calcium hypochlorite) has an LD_{50} value of 850mg/kg of body weight.
DMSO has an LD_{50} value of 14,500mg/kg of body weight.

To compare:

Cooking salt (sodium chloride) has an LD_{50} value of 3,000mg/kg of body weight.
Resochin (chloroquine) has an LD_{50} value of 330mg/kg of body weight.
Lariam (mefloquine hydrochloride) has an LD_{50} value of between 275mg/kg of body weight for guinea pigs and 1,320mg/kg of body weight for a female mouse.

Aspirin (acetylsalicylic acid) has an LD_{50} value of 1,700mg/kg of body weight.
Ibuprofen has an LD_{50} value of 636 mg/kg of body weight.

Tests on other species result in different LD_{50} values per kg of body weight. This means that the LD_{50} values for humans is also almost certainly different. But if we assume for a minute that the human body reacts like that of a rat, a person weighing 70kg would need to take 17.5g of sodium chlorite ($NaClO_2$) in a single dose to produce a 50% likelihood of surviving. Since MMS is supplied in solutions of 28% or 22.4%, you would need to drink at least 62.5ml. It is unlikely that you would succeed. (Sources: http://www.beonlife.eu/forum/3-mms-erfahrungsberichte/38-mmsmiracle-supplement-giftig#38; http://dx.doi.org/10.1002%2Fjat.2550020308; as well as the DMSO safety information leaflet by Serva Elektrophoresis GmbH)

A person weighing 70kg has the same 50% chance of survival (assuming their body reacts like that of a rat) if they consume 210g of cooking salt in one single action, or 23.1g of Resochin. Just as you would not pour huge quantities of salt or tablets down your throat, you should not put large amounts of MMS into your body. The doses recommended by Jim Humble are well below toxic levels. He has established all dose recommendations through testing on himself and on volunteers. Over the course of the last 14 years he has also received thousands of messages containing feedback from people using these substances on their own responsibility, and he has constantly fine-tuned his recommendations as a result.

Synopsis

Here are his safety instructions, which should be observed when handling all these substances:
store sealed in a dry, dark place, out of the reach of children, and at a cool to normal room temperature.

11.1 Handling MMS safely

MMS must be stored in a cool and dark place (i.e. with no direct sunlight). Do not on any account pour a large quantity of pure MMS into a glass or cup. Because it looks like water, there have been instances when it has been drunk by mistake. MMS must be stored out of the reach of children.

If your child has drunk a large quantity of MMS despite these precautions, call a doctor or paramedic. If they have drunk a whole bottle (100

11 • Safety instructions

to 120ml), take them to the hospital's accident and emergency department and tell them that your child has drunk a sodium chlorite solution.

MMS should not be allowed to come into contact with fire or other flammable or explosive substances.

Pure MMS should not be applied to the eyes.

MMS bleaches clothes. If you spill MMS (or MMS dissolved in a small amount of water) on your clothes, rinse with water.

First aid measures
- After inhalation: breathe in fresh air.
- After contact with the skin: wash the skin with soap and water immediately and rinse off thoroughly.
- After contact with the eyes: rinse out the eyes, with eyelids open, for a few minutes under running water and consult a doctor.
- After swallowing: drink as much water as possible to induce vomiting. If available, add half a teaspoonful of sodium bicarbonate to the water. Consult a doctor if in doubt, or if the discomfort persists.

Chlorine dioxide is produced when you activate MMS with acid. At room temperature, chlorine dioxide exists in gas form and it should not be inhaled because it has a poisonous effect when inhaled at high concentrations for long periods. The highest level of concentration allowed in the air at the workplace is $0.1ml \times m^3$, which is equal to 0.1ppm.

This is also approximately the threshold where it can be smelled. So the gas itself warns you with its pungent odour. It does no harm if you can smell a slight chlorine odour for a few seconds. **To handle MMS safely,** it is enough to cover the glass with a saucer during the activation phase or to open a window. Only prolonged exposure to, or deep, direct inhalation of, chlorine dioxide is dangerous to humans. That could be harmful to the eyes or the mucous membrane of the respiratory tract.

Open a window Because the odour is unpleasant and sharp, the chances of inhaling chlorine dioxide by accident are small. If your child should be exposed to chlorine dioxide gas and is showing signs of sickness, have the child examined by a doctor.

The activators citric acid, tartaric acid and hydrochloric acid should also be kept out of the reach of children.

11.2 HANDLING HYDROCHLORIC ACID SAFELY

Hydrochloric acid solutions of 3–9% can be used to activate MMS. Hydrochloric acid solutions below 5% are not classed as dangerous. Beyond that the following applies: do not drink pure hydrochloric acid and do not apply it directly onto the skin or mucous membranes. If it does come into contact with the skin you should rinse thoroughly with water. If your child has swallowed undiluted hydrochloric acid it is advisable to consult a doctor or to go to the hospital.

> General instructions:
> Take off contaminated clothing and dispose of them safely.
> - After inhalation: ensure a plentiful supply of fresh air and place in a resting position.
> - After contact with skin: upon contact with the skin wash off immediately with plenty of water.
> - After contact with eyes: upon contact with the eyes rinse out thoroughly with plenty of water, with eyelids open, and consult an eye specialist.
> - After swallowing: make the person affected drink plenty of water. Do not induce vomiting (there is risk of perforation). Call a doctor immediately.

First aid measures

11.3 HANDLING TARTARIC ACID SAFELY

Undiluted tartaric acid can cause severe eye irritation. A 50% tartaric solution can be used to activate MMS. Tartaric acid is not flammable and does not pose a risk of explosion. It should, however, be stored in a cool place because it decays under thermal exposure. Inhalation can cause slight irritation. Swallowing can lead to irritation of the mucous membranes, nausea and vomiting.

> General instructions:
> Remove clothing contaminated by the product immediately.
> First aiders: consider your own safety. Laypersons should generally not induce vomiting.
> - After inhalation: ensure a plentiful supply of fresh air and consult a doctor as a precaution.

First aid measures

11 • *Safety instructions*

- After contact with skin: rinse off immediately with water. Consult a doctor in case of persisting skin irritation.
- After contact with eyes: rinse out with running water for ten minutes, with eyes open, and consult a doctor.
- After swallowing: rinse out the mouth, and drink a glass of water. Do not induce vomiting. Consult a doctor immediately and show the packaging / label.

11.4 Handling citric acid safely

Citric acid should be stored in a closed container, in a cool, dry place out of the reach of children. Citric acid is an irritant and the eyes are especially sensitive, as are other mucous membranes, and the skin.

First aid measures

- After inhalation: ensure a plentiful supply of fresh air. Consult a doctor if complaints arise.
- After contact with skin: wash off immediately with soap and water.
- After contact with eyes: with eyes open, rinse for 15 minutes under running water and consult a doctor.
- After swallowing: rinse out the mouth and drink plenty of water. Consult a doctor if complaints arise.

Generally speaking, it is unlikely that your child will drink undiluted MMS or activators in large quantities because none of these taste particularly good. If, however, you are worried or are in any doubt, have your child examined by a doctor as a precaution.

11.5 Handling chlorine dioxide solution safely

A 0.3% chlorine dioxide solution does not need to be labelled as a dangerous substance. However, as always, it is the dosage that creates the poison. The following safety instructions should therefore be observed.

First aid measures

- If swallowed, rinse the mouth and drink plenty of water. Consult a doctor if large quantities have been swallowed.

- If large quantities have been inhaled, you should ensure a plentiful supply of fresh air, keep warm, and consult a doctor.

11.6 Handling MMS 2 safely

MMS 2 should be stored in a cool, dry place away from flammable substances. Calcium hypochlorite is available in powder form in capsules as so-called MMS 2.

It is very important to **keep these out of the reach of children**.

If you open the capsules and dissolve the powder in water, an acid forms: hypochlorous acid. If you drink this acid (in the concentration of 400mg, one capsule, in a glass of water) you can cause burns to the mucous membranes. **Follow closely the usage instructions.**

Usage instructions

Drink 2 glasses of water, swallow 1 capsule, drink another glass of water afterwards. The calcium hypochlorite is then only activated by the water in the stomach – and your stomach can handle that. This is the safest way to take it.

If your child somehow gets hold of the calcium hypochlorite, the following first aid measures should be taken.

First aid measures

- After contact with eyes: immediately rinse with clean water for 15 minutes with eyes open. Consult a doctor afterwards.
- After contact with skin: immediately wash off thoroughly with soap and clean water. Take off contaminated clothes immediately and have them washed. Consult a doctor if any irritation persists.
- After swallowing: give nothing to drink and do not induce vomiting. Take to the hospital immediately by ambulance. Never administer anything to an unconscious person.
- After inhalation: go out for fresh air. If breathing irregularly, administer mouth-to-mouth and notify a doctor. If unconscious, place in the recovery position and call an ambulance.

11.7 Handling DMSO safely

Dimethyl sulfoxide, a colourless and odourless liquid, is an irritant and can cause severe eye irritation when applied undiluted onto skin and mucous membranes. DMSO is flammable and must be kept away from sparks, heat, hot surfaces and open flame. It should be stored out of the reach of children in a closed container.

First aid measures
- After inhalation: ensure a plentiful supply of fresh air.
- After contact with skin: wash off immediately with water.
- After contact with eyes: rinse under running water, with eyes open, for a few minutes and consult a doctor.
- After swallowing: rinse the mouth and drink plenty of water.

If in any doubt or if complains persist, consult a doctor.

12

DOSAGE RECOMMENDATIONS FOR PATIENTS WITH VARIOUS ILLNESSES

Please read chapter 6 first if you have not already done so. In that chapter you will find the basic principles of taking MMS explained in detail.

In this chapter I will be describing modified protocols for specific illnesses. The instructions have been compiled from statements made by Jim Humble in his book *Breakthrough*, in the film *Understanding MMS*, and on his various websites. Jim Humble has also sent me previously unpublished material and has given detailed answers to my questions in face-to-face conversations.

The dosage recommendations should not be regarded as medical advice given by me. Since MMS is not approved as a medicine, I cannot prescribe or recommend it. If you decide to experiment with MMS, you do so on your own responsibility. Read the whole book and decide for yourself what conclusions you want to draw from the information contained within. If the illness you suffer from is not specifically listed here, it does not mean that using MMS could not help you too in some way. It simply means that Jim Humble has not published a special dosage recommendation for that illness. You could proceed according to the standard protocol, or consider what other approach would be best for you. Since Jim Humble calls his dosage instructions 'protocols', I have also adopted this term so that it is easier for you to compare when researching his various publications.

AIDS

Activate three drops of MMS in a clean dry glass. After the activation period, top up with water and, if desired, juice (without added vitamin C) and then drink the mixture. Ideally do this eight times a day. If this makes you feel unwell, take just two drops, or even one drop or half a drop. Reduce the number of drops if necessary but do not stop altogether. Increase the dose when you feel better. It is easier to activate 24 drops of MMS in the morning and have it ready to drink, mixed with water and juice, in a closable glass bottle divided into eight equal units. Then drink one-eighth of the content every hour until the bottle is empty, following the new standard protocol (chapter 6).

According to Jim Humble, your chances of becoming well again are good. He writes that it usually takes between 3 days and 3 months to be cured, but usually not more than 30 days. MMS 2 can be given additionally – you will find instructions in chapter 9 'MMS 2'. In some difficult cases, intravenous administration might be required. This should only be carried out by a doctor. See also Jim Humble's book *Breakthrough*, p. 153. All the best!

Allergies

For allergies of all kinds, Jim Humble recommends taking MMS in accordance with the new standard protocol until the complaints have completely abated, and then to take three drops eight times a day for another week. He then recommends switching to a maintenance dose.

If you are still taking antiallergenic drugs when you begin, he recommends leaving three hours before taking MMS, if that is possible. All the best!

Alzheimer's disease

Oxidation of aluminium

As far as I know, only one Alzheimer's patient has been treated with MMS. The treatment was successful, according to the patient's family. I suspect that Alzheimer's patients have a good chance of improving their condition by taking MMS. This is because Alzheimer's is thought to be caused by aluminium – and MMS oxidises metals. Since there is very little experience to go by in this area I would start carefully with the new standard protocol. All the best!

Apoplexy

It is important to act quickly in cases of apoplexy. During the acute stroke, Jim Humble recommends proceeding as follows.

DMSO

Take two level teaspoons of DMSO mixed with at least an equal amount of juice orally every 15 minutes. In addition, take two drops of activated MMS (not mixed with the DMSO) every 15 minutes. You can take or administer the DMSO shortly after the MMS.

After the apoplexy, Jim Humble recommends following the new standard protocol, starting with a quarter of a drop every hour. He also recommends ten drops of DMSO as described above, if damage remains. Please read chapter 10 on DMSO before using it. During this time, the stroke patient should be kept under observation, or at least be asked how they feel at hourly intervals. If they feel better, the dose can be gradually increased, otherwise it is better to take a break. It is, of course, advisable to carry this out under a doctor's supervision. If you are being treated by a homeopathic doctor, he / she should be informed immediately. With so many homeopathic remedies that could do good, I think it is only wise to leave the selection to an experienced colleague who knows you. Self-prescribing homeopathic remedies based on your symptoms is unwise in this case. All the best!

Arteriosclerosis

Jim Humble recommends taking high doses (1–10g) of vitamin C for a number of weeks. Start slowly and reduce the dose if you have diarrhoea. Blood vessel walls need vitamin C for strength and they lose elasticity if there is a lack of vitamin C. The vitamin C displaces the cholesterol to protect the blood vessel walls from collapsing. If they do collapse, the result is an infarction in the affected area. It is therefore wise to first stabilise the blood vessel walls with adequate vitamin C, before removing the deposits. Jim Humble describes one case (in his book *Breakthrough*, p. 156) where a female patient had been told by doctors that her arteries were at least 80% clogged. She took 15 drops of activated MMS three times a day for 30 days. The next time she was tested the degree of obstruction was below 50%. That is a fantastic result after only 30 days, although the dose was fairly high. I would advise taking a more cautious approach, otherwise you can suffer from severe nausea. Avoid that by following the standard protocol and increasing gradually. Jim Humble knows many people who have reduced the calcification of their arteries by using MMS. All the best!

Vitamin C

Arthritis

Jim Humble recommends following the standard protocol, starting with two drops twice a day after meals, and increasing to 15 drops twice a day or three drops eight times a day, if possible.

According to Jim Humble, experience has shown that MMS helps with rheumatoid arthritis and Lyme arthritis but not seronegative arthritis, which is also widespread. This type of arthritis does not show up in blood tests. It is caused by tension and improper use of the muscles, which, in turn, leads to more tension; over the long term this damages the joints. Jim Humble recommends some exercises from the book *Pain Free* by Pete Egoscue with Roger Gittines (Bantam Books, 2000), ISBN 978-0-553-37988-4, or order the DVD *Egoscue Pain Free Workout for Beginners*.

Pete Egoscue claims that pains disappear within a week when doing the exercises, even in serious cases.

I have personally had good experiences with osteopathy and craniosacral therapy. Fortunately, the number of skilled osteopaths and craniosacral therapists has grown significantly over the last 20 years. If the muscles, tendons, fascia or ligaments have contracted severely, undergoing a structural integration such as a SOMA therapy or Rolfing is highly recommended. In some cases that can be very painful, although SOMA therapy is gentler than Rolfing. Alkaline baths can be taken as a preparation since they bring some relief. How painful the treatment is depends mainly on your own resistance. If you succeed in letting go of the resistance, and are able to concentrate on letting go by exhaling, the tension in the muscles abates and so too the pain. This should not surprise you: you produce the muscle tension yourself because of suppressed feelings, the pain of which you do not want to feel consciously. In that moment when you feel, and decide to perceive what is there, the problem can sometimes be solved very quickly. That can, of course, be done without intensive, additional massage (such as with Rolfing or SOMA therapy), but requires excellent concentration and some experience with a form of bodywork: Alexander technique, breath work, bioenergetics, Feldenkrais, qi gong, yoga, zilgrei etc. Have a look to see what is on offer in your area and what you enjoy. It can also be helpful to ask the advice of an experienced physiotherapist.

If you want to do something beneficial for your health, you should choose something that brings you joy, that makes you feel good or that leaves you feeling good afterwards. Then you know it is the right thing for you. Singing in a choir or dancing can also be a pleasant way to help loosen a stiff structure. You will find more ideas in chapter 18 'Guidelines for healthy living'. All the best!

Asthma

Jim Humble recommends taking MMS over a long period of time. It sometimes helps with an acute asthma attack but you should not depend on this. The asthma disappeared in all the patients known to Jim Humble who continued to use MMS until they were able to take 15 drops twice a day for a long period.

His advice is to take two drops twice a day initially (after food) and to increase slowly; and to reduce the dose by two drops if you feel unwell, as stated in the standard protocol. In his book *Breakthrough* (p. 156), Jim Humble tells the story of a woman who took MMS for two months even though the asthma became worse initially. (Author's note: so-called initial aggravations are also known in homeopathy; they sometimes precede a cure.) She persisted for two months and the asthma was completely cured. If you are better able to tolerate smaller doses, try the new protocol: take one-eighth of the daily ration from a large bottle every hour.

If you suffer from asthma, any kind of bodywork could be of great benefit to you. In India asthma is treated with yoga, in China it is treated with qi gong.

Any kind of exercise that helps you to feel freer and more expansive is helpful. You should also think how, through certain thoughts, habits and behavioural patterns, you limit yourself and give away your power. If you observe your feelings when your complaints become more severe, you can make progress through awareness. Do not blame anyone because there is no one to blame, not even yourself. It is not a question of blame but of responsibility. Find out what you need and what is not doing you good, and you can stand up for yourself. No one else can do that for you. If you find it hard to do that then I would advise you to seek a psychotherapist or a therapist who works with kinesiology.

Homeopathy can be very helpful as an accompanying therapy. This list is not compiled in order of priority. See what appeals to you. Or try something quite different, but do something to help yourself. All the best!

Atopic dermatitis

As with other skin diseases, external application of MMS has brought about excellent results. You can use MMS as a spray or in baths. See chapter 8 'More ways of administering MMS'. All the best!

Back pains

You can try any of the protocols you feel suit you best. It often helps, or at least reduces the symptoms. Massage, physiotherapy and SOMA therapy can also bring relief. Careful movement is good in most cases, as are relaxation processes such as autogenic training, craniosacral therapy, osteopathy, zilgrei, singing, music or art therapy. But if the pains persist despite that, it is necessary to become more aware of the source of the pain. When an orthopedic doctor tells you that the pains are the result of a slipped disc that is pressing on a nerve, that is simply a description of your condition at that moment. The origin of the problem lies deeper. Subconsciously, you feel so constrained, under such pressure, that it 'goes on your nerves' in the truest sense of the word. Your body is using the symptom to try to make you aware of the real problem. It is helping you to realise that you are finding it difficult to endure the situation you find yourself in. If such an idea is new to you I encourage you to read chapter 18 'Guidelines for healthy living' carefully.

Usually of psychological origins   Back pain usually has psychological origins. You have taken on too great a load, overstretched yourself, bent yourself out of shape, distorted yourself, or however you want to see it. In her book *Heal Your Body* (Hay House, 2004), ISBN 9780937611357, Louise L. Hay recommends different affirmations for back problems located in different areas of the spine. According to Hay, it is likely that problems in the lumbar spine are caused by fears surrounding money and a lack of financial support. Here is her affirmation to help introduce new thought patterns: 'I trust the process of life. All I need is always taken care of. I am safe.'

She considers old feelings of guilt to be the cause of problems in the thoracic spine and recommends the following affirmation: 'I release the past. I am free to move forward with love in my heart.'

In Louise L. Hay's experience, problems in the cervical spine are caused by a lack of emotional support. Since patients who have tension in the neck musculature often feel unloved and withhold love themselves, she recommends the following affirmation: 'I love and approve of myself. Life supports and loves me.'

Rückenwohl globules   The 'Rückenwohl' energy globules that I have developed also help to support the back. You can buy them individually for the cervical, thoracic, lumbar, sacral, or tailbone area, or all together as a set. If you have suffered chronic pain for years, or if you suffer from wandering pains, I recommend taking the complete set. The energetically imprinted globules have an impact on many levels. That has not been scientifically proven but I have had good results using them.

If you cannot solve your problems by yourself, I recommend you seek guidance from a kinesiologist, psychotherapist or homeopath.

Basal cell carcinoma

In cases of basal cell carcinoma, it is a good idea to apply MMS externally as well as taking it internally.

Activate 20 drops of MMS (ideally with the reduced acid method, see chapter 6.2 'Acid–alkaline balance') in a 60–100ml glass bottle with a spray lid. Add 60ml of water. Spray some of this solution onto the basalioma every one to two hours, but at least twice daily.

You will find the complete protocol for the skin spray in chapter 8 'More ways of administering MMS'. All the best!

Burns

Burns can be life-threatening, depending on their severity and the extent of the affected body area.

You should only treat yourself at home in cases of first- and second-degree burns to small areas of the body. If you are unsure, I urge you to seek medical advice.

Jim Humble has witnessed how MMS has helped with third-degree burns.

In contrast to all other protocols, MMS should be applied to burns undiluted, directly from the bottle. *Undiluted*

You should not add an activator or water in such cases. The faster the MMS is applied to the skin the better.

Spread the solution carefully with the fingertips without pressing on the wound. According to Jim Humble's experience, MMS is a great help and the pain abates within a few seconds, regardless of how large the burn or how bad the wound.

The undiluted MMS solution should only be left on the burn for a maximum of 30 to 60 seconds. Don't bother to look for a clock, just count slowly to 30, then rinse off with clean water. If you cannot find clean water within that time, use any other kind of drinkable fluid as an alternative. **It is very important that the MMS is rinsed off after 30 to 60 seconds at the latest – otherwise the burn will become worse.** *Rinse off quickly*

With serious burns, it is advisable to administer MMS often and to rinse away within 60 seconds each time, as described above. In Jim

Humble's experience, burns can heal in a quarter of the time as a result. The sooner MMS is applied, the more effective the treatment. But applying MMS a few hours later will still bring some benefit.

Make sure that the MMS is rinsed away within one minute, otherwise the condition of the skin will deteriorate.

The homeopathic first aid remedy Cantharis has proved effective in cases of second degree burns. I suggest taking Cantharis 30c every 20 to 30 minutes until the pains are gone, then stop for as long as you remain pain-free. If the pains return, start taking Cantharis 30c again. In cases of third-degree burns, an experienced homeopath should select and prescribe the most appropriate remedy.

It may be advisable or necessary to seek the help of a doctor or to go to hospital, depending on the severity of the burns and regardless of whether or not you treat the burn with MMS or homeopathic remedies. All the best!

For the treatment of **sunburns** see the section on sunburns below.

Cancer

In cases of cancer, I always recommend an alkaline-rich diet or a deacidification regimen since cancer cells thrive in an acidic environment.

See experience reports on pages 68, 70, 72

Jim Humble has received reports from users who have seen their cancers disappear with MMS use, others whose cancers receded, and others who did not see any improvement. His new cancer protocol (as of October 2010) stipulates that you start in the morning with half a drop. If you do not feel unwell take one drop in the evening; the following morning take two drops, then three drops in the evening; the next morning take four drops, and five in the evening, and so on. Increase the number of drops until you reach 15 drops, as long as you continue to feel well. If you feel nauseous, take a break until the nausea has abated and then start again at a dose two drops below the dose that caused the nausea. Stay at that level for a while and then try to increase the dose. If you feel nauseous at half a drop, try to endure the nausea for a few days. If the nausea decreases day by day even though you are continuing to take half a drop once or twice daily, you have the opportunity of working with MMS. You should only increase very slowly, and you should take a certain dose for a few days without experiencing nausea before you increase by half a drop, or later by one drop. If you can tolerate one to two drops, try to increase at a quicker rate, if possible.

Jim Humble's experiences with cancer treatment, even in advanced stages, have led him to recommend the protocol he developed for Stage 4 cancer for all types of cancer:

> *Cancer protocol*
>
> Start with one drop of activated MMS every hour for at least ten hours each day. As always, top up the glass with water and juice if desired (no orange juice). Do not take vitamin C tablets for at least two hours after the last dose. Increase the dose as quickly as possible to eight to ten drops per hour. In advanced stages that will cause nausea. The nausea will only stop when the cancer is no longer there. Increase as quickly as you can and to the degree you can bear. In far advanced stages of cancer, you do not have much time to calmly allow MMS to work without adverse reactions.
>
> Jim Humble recommends taking MMS 2 in addition: see chapter 9 'MMS 2'. Taking MMS hourly in combination with MMS 2 capsules is known as the MMS 2000 protocol. In advanced cancer stages it is advisable to increase as quickly as possible to four to six capsules or more per day. An interval of two hours should be left between two capsules. It is not easy to take MMS 1 and MMS 2 in these quantities. Make sure you don't feel worse taking MMS than without it. MMS 2 should be taken 30 minutes after taking MMS.

Finding the quantity you can tolerate without increasing too slowly or too quickly is a delicate balancing act.

If your body constantly reacts with nausea to even the smallest of quantities and you cannot increase the dose, then MMS is not going to be useful to you.

In such cases, Jim Humble recommends acquiring Indian herbs from Kathleen in Texas. She and her father have been selling these herbs for over sixty years. One vial costs about 60 US$ plus postage (about 40 US$ to Europe, in October 2010). Jim Humble has heard many good things about the effect of these herbs; I have no experience with them. Kathleen can be reached by phone on (001) 806 647 1741 (time difference to Texas: GMT minus 6 hours, UK 17:00 = Texas 11:00). *Indian herbs from Kathleen in Texas*

You may be able to raise your nausea threshold by taking an MMS bath. Read chapter 7 'What to do if adverse reactions occur', or chapter 8 'More ways of administering MMS', for more details on MMS baths.

To assess your healing progress Jim Humble recommends taking a medical cancer test that promises 99% accuracy. The test is called AMAS and it detects the presence of specific cancer antibodies in the blood. Read more on www.oncolabinc.com.

If you have a type of cancer whose progress can be followed by specific tumour markers you can, of course, use these to follow your progress. Discuss this with your doctor.

If your body is able to tolerate small or medium quantities of MMS well, increase slowly. As your nausea threshold rises, you become one step closer to health. If you cannot increase without becoming nauseous, stay at the dose that you can tolerate well. With cancer, you may have to take MMS for a very long time. If it is necessary, and only if you can tolerate it, the most effective treatment is the protocol for advanced stage cancer (Stage 4).

General comments on cancers

It is always helpful to make time for yourself, to look at yourself and to ask why you became ill with an illness that could destroy your physical body. It is also important that you find your own way of dealing with the illness. You will find more ideas in chapter 18 'Guidelines for healthy living' and in the following book recommendations.

Book recommendations for cancer patients

Jim Humble, *Breakthrough: The Miracle Mineral Supplement of the 21st Century* [Fourth Edition], ISBN 978–0982471203

Heinrich Kremer, *The Silent Revolution in Cancer and AIDS Medicine* (Xlibris, 2008), ISBN 978-1436350846

Andreas Moritz, *Cancer is Not a Disease – It's a Survival Mechanism* (Ener-chi.com, 2008), ISBN 978-0976794424

Andreas Moritz, *The Liver and Gallbladder Miracle Cleanse* (Ulysses, 2007), ISBN 978-1569756065

O. Carl Simonton, *Getting Well Again* (Bantam, 1986), ISBN 978-0553172720

Carl Simonton's book is particularly encouraging in that it shows that even so-called terminal patients have become well again by practising the meditation and visualisation exercises. All the best!

Children's diseases

Jim Humble recommends following the new protocol and adjusting the number of drops in accordance with the weight of the child. Further details on this in chapter 6 'How to use MMS'.

Colds

Most types of colds including the common cold are caused by viruses. According to conventional medicine there is no causal treatment. But MMS kills viruses, including rhinoviruses. Depending on specific symptoms, the advice is to start with Clara's 6+6 protocol or with the new standard protocol. Naturopathy can also help in such cases. You can try warm elderberry juice, lime blossom tea, sage tea, warm foot baths, and essential oils to ease swelling of the mucous membranes and to break up secretion (eucalyptus and mountain pine are both suitable to rub in or inhale). However, it is also important to take your body's signals seriously and allow yourself to rest for a few days. Your body would not usually allow the virus to spread unchecked like this; it would eliminate it. If your body does not do that, there must be a reason why. If you caught a real chill then that might well be the cause. But most colds are not caused by the effect of cold weather. Often the real cause is an emotional chill. In such cases some peace and reflection is required. All the best!

Coxsackievirus

Jim Humble's advice is to start cautiously with the standard protocol. If the coxsackie B virus has led to a heart or cardiac valve inflammation, killing the virus may temporarily cause heart palpitations so keep taking low doses until the heart palpitations have abated. **Take care.** All the best!

Diabetes

Jim Humble recommends starting cautiously with the new standard protocol. He knows of many cases where diabetes was cured by MMS but that cannot be guaranteed. If the cells that make insulin have been completely destroyed, MMS cannot cure the diabetes since MMS only kills pathogens and detoxifies the body.

If you want to treat yourself with a higher level of emotional awareness, keep an eye out for ways you deny yourself the sweet things in life and for ways and times where you can enjoy them.

In terms of your diet, stevia may be of interest to you. Stevia and stevioside do not cause an insulin response. Stevioside is even sweeter than stevia. Take care because it is 300 times sweeter than sugar. If you take too much it tastes bitter. You sometimes find stevia in your local supermarket; if not, you will certainly be able to buy it in health food shops and on the internet. Consuming fructose in moderation is also healthy for you. I would advise against consuming refined glucose.

That is certainly not news to you but you may not have known that you can enjoy some sweetness with stevia and still be doing your body a favour. All the best!

Excess weight

A variety of causes can result in excess weight. It can usually be traced back to an unhealthy lifestyle. Read chapter 18 'Guidelines for healthy living'.

Jim Humble recommends starting with two drops of activated MMS and slowly increasing to three drops per 12kg of body weight. Take heed of your individual tolerance threshold and do not overdo it. Some users have had very good results by taking two to six drops, twice to four times a day, continuously for long periods of time. Some lose weight even without changing their dietary habits. However, that does not happen often. If you eat a healthy diet of organic wholefoods, take time to exercise gently in the open air each day, have a balanced psyche and feel at peace with yourself, it may be that you are at the correct weight for you. The study 'Morbidität und Mortalität bei Übergewicht und Adipositas im Erwachsenenalter' [The Morbidity and mortality associated with overweight and obesity in adulthood] (Source: *Deutsches Ärzteblatt*, October 2009, Volume 106, Issue 40), pp. 641–8 revealed that the life expectancy of overweight people is not less than for people of normal weight. The risk of becoming ill with particular diseases is higher, but is the same or even lower for other illnesses. Pronounced obesity does, however, increase both the morbidity and the mortality risk.

In a Finnish study on excess weight and weight loss, Jaakko Kaprio and his colleagues at the University of Helsinki discovered that overweight patients shorten their life expectancy when they lose weight. In total 2,957 people with a body mass index of 25kg/m² or greater took part in the survey.

The participants who, at the start of the study, intended to lose weight and did so increased their risk of dying by 1.86 in comparison to those who had not wanted to lose weight and kept their weight at a stable level. The mortality risk of the first group was even higher than that of the group of participants who did not want to lose weight, and they gained more weight over the period in question. In comparison to the group that kept their weight stable, this group's mortality risk was 1.57 times higher – still lower than the group that lost weight. Because this study was not the first to discover adverse results from weight loss, the Finnish researchers, who were themselves surprised by the significant and unexpected results, see a need for further studies. They suggest testing to see whether the ideal strategy for overweight people is to maintain their weight.

Either way, accepting yourself is the most important precondition for feeling good, which is, in turn, a precondition for achieving and maintaining a healthy weight. *Accepting yourself*

If you are intent on losing weight, here are some reading suggestions:

Leonard Pearson and Lillian Pearson, *The Psychologist's Eat Anything Diet* (Gestalt, 2009), *Reading suggestions*

William L. Wolcott and Trish Fahey, *The Metabolic Typing Diet* (Broadway, 2002)

People with different metabolisms need different foods to lose weight by optimising the metabolism. You will find plenty of books, doctors and alternative practitioners to advise you in this regard if you search using the terms 'metabolic typing' or 'metabolic balancing'. All the best!

Eye diseases

With eye diseases, Jim Humble recommends following one of the internal protocols in addition to applying MMS as an eye drop (see chapter 8.6 'MMS eye drops'). All the best!

Flu (including Swine flu)

These recommendations can probably be used with good results against all new flu types. This protocol was developed to treat Swine flu. Jim Humble was one of the first people in Mexico to fall ill with it. He was admitted to hospital because he was so acutely ill. He continued to take MMS. The doctors treating him were stunned at how quickly he recovered.

(Swine) flu protocol

Start with one drop of activated MMS per hour for three to four hours. **If you do not experience any adverse reactions**, increase to two drops per hour. If you do not feel worse after taking two drops per hour for three or four hours, increase the dose to three drops per hour.

The basic principle is simple. If you do not notice any improvement you need a higher dose. But if you feel worse after taking MMS you should take fewer drops. Remember that you could trigger severe nausea, diarrhoea and vomiting if you take too much. On the other hand, you will also feel worse if the flu gets the upper hand. The aim is to take as many drops as possible every hour without the MMS leading to a deterioration in your general condition. Take as much MMS every hour as you can tolerate for at least eight (ideally twelve) hours a day. Most types of flu disappeared within 24–48 hours when this protocol was used, a little longer with Swine flu. Discontinue the MMS when you feel better. If things do not improve take MMS 2 in addition to the MMS.

The same approach can be used with children, but they should start with a dose of half a drop or less (depending on body weight) and keep a close eye on how your child responds. Take care not to give them too much. If your child feels worse after taking the last MMS dose, take a break or reduce the dose, depending on their condition. You do not normally give a child more than two drops per hour, and never give more than two drops per 23kg of body weight per hour. However, if your child's condition does not improve, the child has probably not been given enough MMS and the flu symptoms are able to advance and develop. The advice, therefore, is not to stay at one drop for too long, but to increase for as long as the child can tolerate it without the MMS causing a reaction. The process is not easy, it requires attentiveness and time. **But at least you have something that kills flu pathogens, something conventional medicine does not have.** In this respect, I know of no safe alternative to this approach as tested by Jim Humble. You can, of course, treat the flu homeopathically if you are in the care of an experienced homeopath who selects the correct remedy. But you will need time and attentiveness with that approach too. The flu is a severe illness in comparison to the common cold which is much more prevalent. It requires careful treatment. If you are in any uncertainty, consult a doctor.

It is certainly a good idea to continue taking MMS **because nothing your doctor can offer you (in December 2010) has the ability to kill the flu virus … but MMS does just that.** All the best!

Heart diseases

The rule with all heart diseases is: the worse your general condition, the more cautiously you should use MMS. It can be helpful to start slowly with foot baths or with less than one drop internally in accordance with the new standard protocol, and then increase in small steps if you tolerate it well. If you do not tolerate MMS well when using the new standard protocol, you could switch to slow activation based on the Fischer method.

In cases of inflamed cardiac valve diseases, killing the bacteria can lead to temporary heart palpitations. That usually passes after a few days. All the best! *Temporary heart palpitation*

Hepatitis A, B, C, and other hepatitis types

Since the function of the liver will be impaired due to the inflammation, it is particularly important to start cautiously. Jim Humble recommends starting with two drops because most people tolerate two drops as a first dose. I would rather start with one drop and increase to two drops at the second dose. This is because once severe nausea has set in, there is a danger that you can develop a strong aversion to taking the doses. The aim is to increase the number of drops slowly until you have reached three drops eight times a day, or 15 drops twice a day. A gentler approach to dosing is to activate the quantity you plan to take over the day in the morning, and then drink this in eight units at hourly intervals. Jim Humble has discovered that most people are able to tolerate an even and continuous intake, better than they are able to tolerate a high dose once or twice a day. He sets 24 drops as a target for the day, to be activated in the mornings. You can, of course, start lower and increase later. *Start very slowly*

You should be under the care of a doctor and have your liver values tested at reasonable intervals. Make sure you drink enough water and support your liver through detoxification (see chapter 7 'What to do if adverse reactions occur'). All the best! *Drink plenty of water*

Herpes

See images and experience report on pages 61-2

In severe cases, Jim Humble recommends following the new standard protocol for several days. In more moderate cases start with one drop eight times a day, increasing each day until you are taking three drops eight times a day. You should do this for at least a week. If you still see no significant improvement, Jim Humble advises increasing to 4 to 6 drops up to ten times a day. If that is still not enough to bring about an improvement he administers MMS 2. However, in his experience the new standard protocol is more than enough in most cases of herpes. It is sometimes necessary to continue treatment for two to three months in persistent cases. Using an MMS skin spray alongside internal doses is usually beneficial (see chapter 8.1).

Herpes, especially herpes zoster, is a serious illness that shows that your physical system is completely overburdened. Reduce the stress in your life and look after yourself. Read chapter 18 'Guidelines for healthy living'. All the best!

High blood pressure

Jim Humble recommends following the new protocol. There are cases in which MMS helped to normalise blood pressure. The root cause of blood pressure is usually of an emotional nature. That, of course, means that conventional medicine cannot find the cause. And how could it by measuring physical parameters while the cause is almost certainly to be found in suppressed emotions? Treating high blood pressure is therefore a difficult business. But it is always better to start the journey than to do nothing at all. I recommend you read chapter 18 'Guidelines for healthy living'. All the best!

HIV, *see* AIDS

Hypertension, *see* High blood pressure

Injuries

Depending on the severity of the injury, it may be necessary to seek the advice of a doctor or to go to hospital. MMS has been used to treat a wide range of injuries. Activated MMS is very useful to rinse deep wounds. If possible, a surgeon or casualty specialist should carry this out, or a GP if trained in such methods. Four drops of activated MMS in 10ml of water have been successfully used to rinse wounds.

With superficial injuries it is advisable to apply MMS regularly, using a spray bottle. See chapter 8 'More ways of administering MMS'.

Homeopathic remedies can be used to treat injuries with great effect. The standard remedy for injuries of all kinds is Arnica. You can give the 30c potency as first aid for most injuries. Higher potencies are necessary for more serious injuries such as brain trauma. However, these must only be prescribed by an experienced homeopath. I always have some Arnica 30c with me in my homeopathic travel kit, in my car, and of course at home. I recommend keeping a bottle of Arnica in your bag so that you always have some at hand in an emergency, for example if a child falls. Arnica helps by resolving mental shock as well as by giving the physical body the signals it needs to start organising the healing process as quickly as possible following injuries of all kinds.

Staphysagria is the main remedy for cuts. Hypericum is indicated for nerve injuries. Rhus tox usually helps with pulled and sprained muscles.

Homeopathic remedies work mainly by providing the body with information. It is, therefore, not the quantity taken that determines the effect, but rather the potency and the frequency of administration. In cases of non-life-threatening injuries, the 30c potency is perfect. Take a dose every few minutes to every few hours, depending on the pains. **If you feel better, stop taking it until you notice a deterioration.**

If the healing process is slow and protracted, I recommend the globule tube 'Gute Regeneration' [Good Regeneration] from the energy globules set. See www.informierteGlobuli.de.

Lyme disease

In Jim Humble's experience, healing this illness can be a long-drawn-out process. He recommends starting with a dose of one drop of activated MMS per hour and increasing as soon as possible, if necessary up to six drops per hour for at least ten hours a day. By proceeding in this way, a significant amelioration of complaints was observed in some cases within a few weeks. Some cases required treatment for months or even years. These days, Jim Humble recommends starting with the new standard protocol to avoid adverse reactions and increasing as you see fit – that is, as quickly as possible but as slowly as necessary.

Users who did not initially see any improvements at all have sometimes had good results after increasing the dose – as far as that was possible. In some circumstances, however, they have to take MMS continuously for years.

If your nausea threshold is very low, an MMS bath may help. Jim Humble recommends taking hot baths with at least 15 drops of activated MMS a number of times a week. If the illness is very persistent, he recommends taking MMS 2 in addition to the MMS.

I know people who have noticed an improvement in their Lyme symptoms after only a short time. If you are not one of those people I recommend you read chapter 18 'Guidelines for healthy living'.

In terms of emotional imbalances which allow illnesses to take root, it is suspected that Lyme disease may involve a deep-seated lack of love for oneself or even self-hatred. If you want to begin to change that, it is usually necessary to have some help from outside, for example through homeopathy, psychotherapy, kinesiology, faith healing or other treatments. It is best to choose an approach with which you feel a connection and find someone with a good reputation.

Many roads lead to the same goal, and anyone you warm towards is right for you at this time; we may all need different things. But going it yourself is not likely to work. I am not saying that it is impossible, only not very likely. This is because if you held the key to your problems, you would not have repressed your consciousness so deeply that you became chronically ill as a result. If you think that looking for help, and accepting it, is worthwhile then that is a very promising start. All the best!

Malaria

For malaria, Jim Humble always recommends a dose of 15 drops of activated MMS, to be repeated one or two hours later. Malaria patients have been completely cured within 24 hours in almost all cases. If the patient is still not completely well, Jim Humble suspects that another disease is present, in addition to the malaria. He then recommends taking a third dose of 15 activated drops of MMS plus a dose of MMS 2.

Please observe the special procedure for administering MMS 2 (see chapter 9).

Remarkable success The treatment of malaria is, as far as Jim Humble has been able to observe, a story of absolute success. In Africa, the ordinary village dwellers have neither the money nor the means to have laboratory tests carried out. They feel well and go home. That was the case with 100% of the malaria patients treated by Jim Humble. He had laboratory tests carried out for documentation purposes in his own case and in that of 100 other patients. After taking MMS, no malaria pathogens could be detected in the blood of any of the test persons, without exception.

It is a great blessing that in future, when MMS becomes well known, malaria patients will have a safe, simple, cheap and sustainable method of treatment.

Those travelling to the tropics could also switch to a healthier alternative to conventional malaria prophylaxis with their range of side effects. All the best!

Melanoma

As with other skin cancers, the following approach has proved useful for melanomas (in addition to internal use).

Put 20 drops of MMS in a (60 to 100ml) glass bottle with a spray lid. The reduced acid method of activation is preferable (see chapter 6.2 'Acid–alkaline balance').

When the activation is complete, pour 60ml of water into the glass bottle. Spray the MMS solution onto the melanoma every one to two hours. Wash off with clear water after three to five minutes, or just before spraying the next dose of MMS.

You will find details of the skin spray protocol in chapter 8 'More ways of administering MMS'. I recommend you read the general remarks on cancers, as well as chapter 18 'Guidelines for healthy living'. All the best!

MRSA

MRSA is the abbreviation for methicillin-resistant Staphylococcus aureus, sometimes known as multiple-resistant Staphylococcus aureus. The Staphylococcus aureus bacterial infection is among the infections most often caught in hospitals worldwide. Conventional medical treatment becomes difficult when a strain of bacteria develops a resistance to methicillin and other antibiotics, an increasingly familiar scenario over the last few years.

Conventional medicine has at its disposal only a small number of expensive medicines that come with a number of side effects. Every severe MRSA infection leads to a significant increase in mortality and costs an average of between 6,000 and 20,000 euros.
(Source: information leaflet by the Centre of Excellence for Patient Safety in cooperation with the Association of Statutory Health Insurance)

Symptoms The following symptoms can arise with an MRSA infection: general skin infections such as carbuncles, furuncles, abscesses, styes, osteomyelitis, meningitis, endocarditis, pneumonia, flu-like symptoms such as high fever, nausea, vomiting, eruptions on the skin of the hands and feet, headaches, pain in the limbs and back muscles, blood poisoning, septic arthritis, septic shock ...

Probability of death According to Jim Humble, the statistical probability of death lies somewhere between 11% and 80%. It is 80% when untreated, 11% when you have the weakest strain of Staphylococcus and receive the standard treatment. Jim Humble says that MMS has a curative effect in 99% of cases. Chlorine dioxide certainly has the power to kill all kinds of bacteria – including MRSA.

Jim Humble's MRSA treatment consists of two measures.

Internal use Step 1: follow the new standard protocol – MMS 1000 protocol – and increase the dose until you have reached three drops per hour.

Step 2: you will need a clean, dry, see-through glass with a diameter that is big enough to fit over the running sore or the affected area. Use smaller glasses for smaller sores.

External use Put six drops of MMS in the glass and add the corresponding number of drops of activator. Swirl the glass to mix the liquids. A yellow chlorine dioxide gas will now form. Hold the opening of the glass over the affected area of skin or hold the affected area of skin over the glass, in a manner in which no liquid touches the skin but that allows the chlorine dioxide gas to come into contact with the skin. The chlorine dioxide gas can now penetrate the area of skin infected by the MRSA and tackle the sore. Leave the glass on the same spot for a maximum of five minutes – no longer than that, otherwise it can damage the skin and it takes longer to heal. If you remove the glass in time (before 5 minutes have passed), you usually achieve a pain-free reduction in the infection. If the MRSA is still not completely destroyed after one treatment you can repeat the procedure after 4 hours but not before, otherwise it burns the skin. Depending on your sensitivity you can damage the skin slightly, even in less than five minutes. However, the skin will heal within a short period of time. If you have sensitive skin you can reduce the intensity of skin irritations by leaving a gap between the edge of the glass and your skin so that some of the chlorine dioxide gas can escape.

You can treat all areas of skin affected by MRSA with this same five-minute treatment. It is not painful. Following the chlorine dioxide gas treatment, it is advisable to cover the treated area with Vaseline and a bandage.

Jim Humble has been treating MRSA patients for a long time. The patients were cured within periods ranging from one week to two months, but usually within a few weeks.

Multiple sclerosis (MS)

There have been reports of improvements in cases of MS treated with MMS, but never a cure.

I recommend following the new standard protocol, increasing as your level of tolerance allows and combining with external application. It is certainly worth giving it a try since the options offered by conventional medicine are very limited for MS. There is a variety of helpful methods available to MS patients: most ameliorate symptoms, but not everything helps everyone. Treatments that are especially suited to MS include reflexology, Feldenkrais, hippotherapy, or cold therapy. Classical homeopathy offers the possibility of a cure in the sense that the progression of the disease can be stopped if the correct remedy is chosen. But even with homeopathy, damaged tissue can only be regenerated to a limited extent. All the best!

Parkinson's disease

There are reports of improvements in Parkinson's patients, but no reports of outright cures. Jim Humble recommends following the new standard protocol and increasing the dose depending on tolerance. It might also be beneficial to combine this approach with external application. All the best!

Severe illnesses

The most severe illnesses should be treated by a doctor. Jim Humble recommends following the protocol for the last stages of cancer. See 'Cancer'.

He has, with success, advised a number of patients whose doctors had given up hope. Even when a patient is beyond treatment in the eyes of conventional medicine, he still believes there is hope for improvement or even a cure if it is possible to follow the MMS 2000 protocol. All the best!

Skin cancer

Jim Humble's recommendation for skin cancer is to spray MMS on the area every one to two hours. In some cases the skin condition changed within a few days. The cancer first shrivelled and later fell off. However, he recommends taking the MMS orally at the same time, in accordance with the new standard protocol. In persistent cases, Jim Humble recommends applying DMSO to the skin after spraying it with MMS.

It is essential that you read chapter 10 on DMSO beforehand. All the best!

See images and experience reports on page 72

Skin diseases of all kinds

Skin diseases usually respond well to MMS sprays or MMS baths. See chapter 8 'More ways of administering MMS'. All the best!

Sleep disorders

MMS can sometimes be very helpful. I recommend taking ten drops of activated MMS in water (if you can tolerate it) in the evenings. It is best to start by taking two drops and then increasing every day to see where your tolerance threshold lies. Here is a good exercise from the field of kinesiology to help you fall asleep: place one hand on your navel and the other on your forehead. It makes no difference which hand is above and which is below. After 10 to 15 minutes, the energies in these areas should have become balanced and you will hopefully have fallen asleep. If not, take a deep breath and switch the hands. Make sure that you are lying comfortably. I have developed energetically imprinted globules for people who find it difficult to calm down, to fall asleep and to sleep through the night. You can buy them via my website www.informierte Globuli.de. Since users do not always achieve the desired results with the globules, they come with a six-week right of return.

The basis for healing sleep disorders should be a regular, rhythmic lifestyle, daily movement in fresh air, and calming herbal teas. If during the day you repeatedly overexert yourself, become agitated and overstimulate your body, it is a bit much to ask it to fall asleep at the touch of a button. It is also helpful to avoid becoming upset or irritated regarding your lack of sleep when you are awake. The stress hormones released if you do will certainly keep you awake. If nothing helps, I advise you to seek help from a homeopath or a kinesiologist. Acupuncture could also be helpful in the short term in that it harmonises the chi, especially the liver energy. You might also want to learn autogenic training, qi gong, tai chi or yoga so that you are better at bringing yourself into a calm state. All the best!

Stomach ulcers

MMS has also helped with stomach ulcers. Jim Humble recommends starting cautiously with one drop or less (you can get less than one drop by diluting it even more in accordance with the new standard protocol). If you are unsure, I recommend starting with foot baths and increasing slowly (see chapter 8.5 'MMS foot baths'), or slow activation based on the Fischer method. All the best!

Stroke, *see* Apoplexy

Sunburn

Put the undiluted solution without activator on the burned areas of skin, as with burns – a sunburn is, after all, a type of burn. Put plenty of undiluted MMS directly from the bottle onto the sunburned areas and spread with the fingertips or with a clean towel. Allow the MMS to work for 15 to 30 seconds before rinsing the solution off thoroughly with plenty of water. No traces of MMS should be left on the skin, otherwise the burn will deteriorate. You have a five minute window in which to rinse the MMS away thoroughly. Depending on the extent and severity of the burns, it may be necessary to consult a doctor.

Prevention is better than cure. Avoid sunbathing for long periods, especially on the first few days of a holiday at the seaside or in the mountains. It is better to stay in the shade, or to keep sensitive areas covered. Applying huge quantities of sunscreen is not healthy because of the chemicals and metals that such products contain. All the best!

Swine flu, *see* Flu

Tinnitus

According to an old Chinese saying, Traditional Chinese Medicine (TCM) considers ringing in the ears to be the result of a lack of kidney yin. If the ringing has started recently, I recommend rest as a first measure. Kidney energy is exhausted through overwork, excitement, anger, lack of sleep or lack of water. Secondly, drinking enough water is of fundamental importance. See my remarks on water and salt in chapter 18 'Guidelines for a healthy life'.

Rest

Water

If tinnitus or hearing loss has set in then the body has shown you the red card. I advise you to drink about five litres of water (for an adult weighing about 70kg) for the next few weeks. Together with water and rest, MMS can be helpful. It is best to start with the new standard protocol. I have also seen very good results with acupuncture and qi gong exercises. If you are fostering old resentments, you should seek advice from a kinesiologist, psychotherapist or homeopath. If you fail to resolve your resentments, your kidney energy will not be able to replenish itself. All the best!

Resolve old resentments

MMS FOR HEALTHY PEOPLE

If you enjoy excellent health you can still benefit from taking MMS as a way of maintaining your level of well-being.

Jim Humble recommends that healthy people start with one drop and increase slowly to find a dose they can tolerate without experiencing adverse reactions. Read chapter 6 'How to use MMS' if you have not already done so.

Whenever we say that you should take one drop (or however many drops), we mean one drop of MMS + activator, then wait for the activation period to pass before topping up with water.

Take only what you can tolerate. Increase to 15 drops twice a day. If you cannot tolerate that, stay below your nausea threshold and take the quantity you can tolerate twice a day or multiple times a day without experiencing adverse reactions. Jim Humble considers 8 drops three times a day as the optimal approach.

Only take what you can tolerate

Many people who can only tolerate small quantities of MMS find that it helps to take MMS baths because detoxification occurs via the skin, taking the burden off the liver. See chapter 8 'More ways of administering MMS'.

If you can tolerate 15 drops of MMS twice a day, take that dose for a week. Alternatively you can take 3 to 4 drops eight times a day. Both these doses are usually only possible after increasing slowly, otherwise most people experience nausea or diarrhoea. To test this, start with one drop per hour and, if you can tolerate that, increase to two drops and so on until you reach a maximum level of 3 drops eight times a day (for adults of 70kg). If at any point you experience adverse reactions, take a break until they pass, then restart at a reduced dose and do not increase for at least 14 days. If you have adverse reactions when taking just one drop, activate one drop and put it in a bottle that you can divide into eight equal units. Then fill the bottle with water, and juice if desired. Take the dose of your choice, for example one-eighth of a drop every hour. The same is true when you take more drops, up to an ideal dose of 24 drops per day. After a week at 15 drops twice a day or 3 drops eight times a day you can assume that your body is free of toxins, heavy metals, yeast, fungi and microorganisms.

Maintenance dose   At that stage, switch to the so-called maintenance dose. Jim Humble used to recommend eight drops twice a week or six drops five times a week. In his view, this reduces the chances of falling ill with acute illnesses, such as flu or other infections, by 95%. Today, he recommends that people up to the age of 60 take six drops twice a week and those older than 60 take six drops daily as a maintenance dose.

Taking a continuous maintenance dose can be compared to tending your garden. If weeds are removed immediately, they do not have time to develop and spread. Applied to the human organism, that means that invading pathogens or poisons are immediately eliminated or made harmless by MMS before they can become established and spread in the body. This increases your chances of staying fit and healthy. Jim Humble recommends taking a maintenance dose for the rest of your life for this very reason.

In my experience, this approach suits about 90% of people, of whom only about 50% will be able to tolerate the dose of 15 drops twice a day. So it is possible that you will only be able to tolerate ten drops once a day but that your body is able to cleanse itself completely despite that, if you keep it up for three months. For example, if you can only tolerate three drops a day your body will need more time: at three drops, about 13 months; at five drops, about eight months; at eight drops, about seven months. I have arrived at these figures through kinesiological testing and they serve as a point of orientation. The required cleansing period at a certain number of drops can be longer or shorter for different individuals because we are all different and have different processes under way. The (tested) figures stated refer to what most users require to have a high probability of ensuring that pathogens are eliminated and the problem of heavy metal poisoning is addressed.

About 13% (tested) require less MMS to achieve the same result. It is best that you find out for yourself whether, and in what way, and at what dose, you should administer MMS for your own personal benefit.

Even sensitive persons who only tolerate small amounts of MMS can, in most cases, cleanse their body if they proceed cautiously and give their body time.

According to my kinesiological testing, it is advisable for sensitive persons to switch to a maintenance dose of two drops twice a week afterwards.

You will have noticed that there is a huge difference between the recommended doses here. Some people become terribly nauseous from taking just a couple of drops while others can tolerate single doses of 18 drops without adverse reactions. You will probably find that you are between these two poles.

If you are healthy and want to take MMS as a preventative measure or as a means of detoxification, the best way to find out how much MMS you can tolerate is by starting with one drop and increasing slowly. If you become nauseous, take a break until you feel better and then start again at a reduced dose, for example take half the dose that you tolerate well and increase again slowly, staying at each dosage level for a few days before increasing. In this way, you will discover the best way to make MMS work for you without triggering a negative effect.

If you want to reduce the MMS dose after having cured an illness with it, you know how much MMS you can tolerate and what dose was conducive to your health. As I have said, there are people who quickly experience a significant improvement in their condition even at small doses. I suggest the following: if you needed a large dose of MMS to recover from an illness (16 drops or more), follow Jim Humble's maintenance protocol. If you did not need that much for your health to improve, a lower maintenance dose is probably enough for you. That might be anywhere from three drops three times a week to four drops five times a week. My kinesiology tests indicate that two drops twice a week is enough for some particularly sensitive people.

You must decide for yourself whether or not you want to use MMS as a preventative measure and at what dose. The stated dosage recommendations are for information only and serve as a point of orientation. They do not represent a prescription.

14

MMS FOR ANIMALS

A number of people who have experienced good results when using MMS on themselves have given it to their sick pets, for example when they have an infection, or to deworm. Dogs, cats and horses, in particular, have been successfully treated with MMS. It seems likely that MMS could be used on all mammals. Dairy and livestock farmers could all benefit from this information since MMS does not leave any harmful products in the body. These recommended doses have been compiled by Jim Humble and Lothar Paulus based on their experience and on reports by animal owners. They do not represent a prescription in a veterinary sense. The same rule is true when treating animals as when treating yourself: you take full responsibility for treatment because MMS has been approved only for use as a water steriliser and not as a medicine.

If you have not read the general guidelines on the use of MMS, please read chapter 6 'How to use MMS' first.

When treating animals, the following guidelines apply.

Observe closely Observe your animals closely. Only then will you notice how much MMS they need, or are able to tolerate. If you only notice that the dose is too high when the animals begin to suffer from diarrhoea, the effort and work required then will be disproportionally greater than if you had watched them closely to see how they progress, and what mood they are in. Some animals tolerate significantly higher doses of MMS per kg of body weight than humans. If there are no signs of improvement in an animal suffering from an infection, it is usually advisable to increase the dose hourly until there are clear signs that the animal is getting better. If in doubt, consult a veterinarian. Some animals quickly suffer from diarrhoea, but each individual case is different. That can, of course, be part of the cleansing process that leads to a cure, but it should be avoided if at all possible. It is best to start with a low dose and then increase quickly or slowly depending on the level of urgency.

MMS can be administered very easily with a single-use syringe without a needle. Draw the activated MMS diluted with water into the syringe and inject it into the animal's mouth.

Dosage recommendations for small animals

For small animals, it is advisable to use the weaker MMS solution especially produced for animals below 12kg (3.5% sodium chlorite). It is easier to administer in smaller doses, and it is easier to find the tolerance threshold.

- **Starting dose for an animal of about 1.5kg:**
  1 drop of MMS (sodium chlorite 3.5%) and 1 drop of activator (10% citric acid)
- **For an animal of about 3kg:**
  2 drops of MMS (sodium chlorite 3.5%) and 2 drops of activator (10% citric acid)
- **For an animal of about 6kg:**
  4 drops of MMS (sodium chlorite 3.5%) and 3 drops of activator (10% citric acid)
- **For an animal of about 9kg:**
  6 drops of MMS (sodium chlorite 3.5%) and 4 drops of activator (10% citric acid)
- **For an animal of about 12kg:**
  8 drops of MMS (sodium chlorite 3.5%) and 5 drops of activator (10% citric acid)

Larger animals can be given MMS in the same concentrations as humans. In one example, 10% citric acid was given as the activator. You can, of course, use 50% citric acid, 50% tartaric acid, or 3–9% hydrochloric acid as an activator. The quantities must then be reduced accordingly.

Dosage recommendations for larger animals

- **Starting dose for an animal of about 12 to 24kg:**
  1 drop of MMS (sodium chlorite 22.4%) and 5 drops of activator (10% citric acid)
- **For an animal of about 24 to 36kg:**
  2 drops of MMS (sodium chlorite 22.4%) and 10 drops of activator (10% citric acid)
- **For an animal of about 36 to 48kg:**
  3 drops of MMS (sodium chlorite 22.4%) and 15 drops of activator (10% citric acid)

- **For an animal of about 48 to 52kg:**
  4 drops of MMS (sodium chlorite 22.4%) and 20 drops of activator (10% citric acid)
- **For an animal of 52kg and more:**
  5 drops of MMS (sodium chlorite 22.4%) and 25 drops of activator (10% citric acid)

If your animal tolerates that well you can increase up to a maximum of 15 drops twice a day, or in serious cases, 4 drops eight times a day at hourly intervals.

If your animal suffers from diarrhoea after a dose, or shows any other signs of intolerance, you should take a break until all adverse reactions have abated. Then restart at a reduced dose: ideally one to two drops below the last dose that was tolerated well. This dose can then be maintained for a long period of time. It is the same for both animals and humans alike.

Tips

Here are further tips based on the experience reports.
- Horses: put MMS in wheat bran. They can smell it in oats and will refuse to eat it.
- Dogs: dripped onto bread and wrapped around a sausage.
- Bees: add 18 drops of activated MMS per 10kg bee food.
- Calves: give them 20 drops of activated MMS to drink in a litre of milk. Caution! According to Andreas Kalcker, MMS causes diarrhoea if, because of the calf's age or method of swallowing, it enters the calf's rumen instead of the true stomach (abomasum). MMS must immediately be discontinued in such cases.
- Doves: put six drops of MMS in four litres of water to drink continuously – it takes about 14 days for them to become familiar with it.

MMS spray for eye and ear diseases in animals

Activate four drops of MMS, ideally following the reduced-acid method. When the activation period has passed, add 100ml of water and pour the solution into a glass bottle with a spray lid. Spray the MMS solution onto the animal's eyes or ears. Repeat as required.

In cases of severe infections, halve the quantity of water to 50ml so that the spray is twice as strong.

VITAMIN C AND OTHER ANTIOXIDANTS

Antioxidants are used in the human body to capture free radicals, to reduce substances that have an oxidative effect, and to chelate metal ions, as well as for many other processes. For example, the presence of vitamin C in the stomach prevents nitrite and secondary amines from forming cancer-causing nitrosamines.
(Source: see 'UGB: Vitamine C – Viel hilft viel? (1)' [Vitamin C – the more the merrier?] http://ugb.de/e_n_1_140758_n_n_n_n_n_n_n.html)

MMS should not be taken together with large amounts of vitamin C or other powerful antioxidants.

The reason for this is obvious. Since chlorine dioxide rids the body of pathogens and poisons through oxidisation, the presence of antioxidants would be disruptive. As the name suggests, they have an *antioxidant* effect, which means that they neutralise the effect of oxidation. Chlorine dioxide has the capacity to steal electrons from pathogens, while antioxidants donate electrons. If the two come together they will neutralise each other and neither one is of any use to the body. In principle, both the MMS and the antioxidant can be very beneficial to the body, but not if both are administered at the same time. The (interfering) effect of antioxidants is dependent on quantity. Jim Humble recommends adding apple or other fruit juices (except orange juice) to the MMS mixture to improve its taste. Apple juice contains vitamin C, but not in high enough quantities to significantly reduce the effect of MMS. However, if the juice contains artificially added vitamin C, or if orange juice is used, the quantity of vitamin C is too high and it neutralises the effect of MMS temporarily or completely. That is also true of nutritional supplements that contain antioxidants, especially vitamin C tablets. These should never be taken within two hours before or after taking MMS and ideally you should leave an interval of four hours. In the long term it is wise to take plenty of vitamin C or other antioxidants. If you only take MMS once a day, for example in the evenings, you can take vitamin-rich nutrients containing high levels of antioxidants without

Antioxidants neutralise the effect of MMS

15 • Vitamin C and other antioxidants

Take vitamins at different times

impeding the effect of MMS. Or you can take MMS in the morning and supplement your vitamins in the afternoon and evening. Most people digest fruit and vegetables, including salads, better before 5 p.m.; many people cannot digest raw foods properly in the evening, which can lead to fermentation and flatulence. If you are able to digest raw foods in the evening, continue in that way. If you are taking MMS in small doses at hourly intervals eight times a day from the morning onwards because of a serious illness, it is recommended that you take your vitamins two to four hours after the last dose of MMS. Alternatively, you could take a break of a few days after taking MMS for a few weeks, or take MMS just once a day in the evening, and during this period take plenty of vitamins during the day. Pay attention to how you feel and do not overtax your body. Oxidative work is strenuous for the body and taking a break every now and again can be a wise choice. It all depends on your condition. If you pay attention to how you feel, you will know how much is right for you. It is just as important to take the correct amount of antioxidants as it is MMS: too much can be just as harmful as too little.

If you use naturally available antioxidants it is unlikely that you will overdose. Antioxidants are available in higher concentrations in nutritional supplements. Generally, I do not consider taking these to be a good idea since this can easily lead to overdoses of vitamin E in particular. It can be a good idea for some individuals with increased needs to take antioxidant supplements. An increased need usually arises in cases of protracted, chronic illnesses. If you want to supplement your diet with antioxidants for this reason I advise the following:

- between 6 a.m. and 9 a.m.: a vitamin-rich breakfast with plenty of fruit and the nutritional supplement of your choice (ideally one which is as natural as possible)
- about 10 a.m. to 11 a.m.: a fruit snack if desired
- between noon and 1 p.m.: vitamin-rich lunch with plenty of vegetables
- between 3 p.m. and 11 p.m.: hourly doses of MMS following the new standard protocol
- about 6 p.m.: dinner

It is important for your health that you maintain a vitamin-rich diet even if you are supplementing with antioxidants.

Vitamin C and other antioxidants

A natural diet is important simply because we cannot be sure that we humans have discovered all the substances that a natural food contains. It may be that certain individual substances have not yet been discovered. So if you are taking a vitamin complex something may still be missing. There are substances in a piece of fruit that scientists have isolated and there are probably others that are yet to be discovered. When you eat the fruit, these substances are all absorbed together and have a synergistic effect. Since we do not know whether or not something is missing when we take synthetic products, and if so what, it is preferable to use antioxidants from natural sources.

It can be the case that certain isolated substances cannot be fully absorbed by the body on their own because other substances must be present for them to be properly utilised.

Nature provides everything that is necessary for life. I therefore recommend trying to meet your antioxidant requirements by eating foods that are as natural as possible.

Natural foods

> Citrus fruits, kiwi fruit, acai berries, acerola, sea buckthorn, redcurrants, rosehips, spinach, bell peppers and potatoes are **high in vitamin C**. Nuts and sunflower seeds are **high in vitamin E**. Palm oil and various other oils are rich in tocotrienol, which is a member of the vitamin E family. Choose oils that have been produced in a way that conserves the nutrients. Many vitamins are lost when oils are heated and the same is true for fruit and vegetables. You will find other antioxidants in garlic, wine, tea and coffee.

Natural sources of vitamin C

Quantity is the decisive factor when consuming stimulants. You do yourself no favours by overindulging. How much agrees with you is purely an individual matter and can be subject to your respective biorhythms, or changes as a result of age. There is no right or wrong in any absolute sense.

You should always find out for yourself what – and how much – is good for you. The foods and stimulants listed above are not comprehensive. They are intended merely as a point of orientation.

Your body produces its own antioxidants: proteins such as transferrin, albumin, ceruloplasmin, hemopexin and haptoglobin, as well as enzymes such as superoxide dismutase, glutathione peroxidase, catalase, and others.

Your body has an intelligent system at its disposal which allows it to

15 • Vitamin C and other antioxidants

produce more or less antioxidants, as required. It is all wonderfully regulated if only we allow nature's wisdom to work.

If your body has become so far out of balance that you are now suffering from an illness, it is helpful to support it in terms of oxidation as well as by providing sufficient antioxidants, because it needs both. However, they should not be given at the same time, but rather alternated according to a suitable timetable. After all, you wouldn't want to sleep and go jogging at the same time, would you?

16

FURTHER INFORMATION ON MMS

If you wish to know more about MMS, the following media sources might interest you:

1. Books

Jim Humble, *Breakthrough: The Miracle Mineral Supplement of the 21st Century* (Parts 1 and 2, Fourth Edition), ISBN: 978-0982471203
This is the original book by Jim Humble.

Jim Humble, *The Master Mineral Solution of the Third Millennium* (Osmora, 2011)
Jim Humble's latest e-book.

Leo Koehof, Jim Humble and Dr Wolfgang Storch, *MMS: An Easy Cure* (Jim Humble Publishing, 2012)
Leo Koehof writes about his journeys with Jim Humble in Africa and Europe, and about his experiences using MMS. Some of the reports are very moving and illustrate clearly what MMS can do.

Leo Koehof, *MMS: Pros and Cons* (Jim Humble Publishing, 2011), ISBN 978-9088790287

Jim Humble's training seminar (in English) can be ordered as a home study course by email from the following address:
genesis2mission@gmail.com

2. DVD

MMS Verstehen / Understanding MMS (Daniel-Peter Verlag)
If you want to watch the people mentioned in this book talking 'live'

about MMS, then I can recommend this DVD. Over 105 minutes, the topic of MMS and chlorine dioxide is examined and explained in detail using informative graphics and fascinating interviews. You come to know Jim Humble, the physician Dr John Humiston, the chemist Professor Antonio Romo Paz, and a number of MMS users. Now in its fourth print run, and including a 16-page booklet with interesting articles (in German only) on MMS. The DVD audio can be set to English, German or Spanish. ISBN 978-3981291704 www.daniel-peter-verlag.de

3. Internet

ENGLISH WEBSITES:

www.jimhumble.biz
Jim Humble's MMS homepage

www.bioredox.mysite.com
Thomas Lee Hesselink's homepage

www.miraclemineral.org
You can download the first part of Jim Humble's *Breakthrough* book free of charge, and download the second part for a fee. You can also order the DVD *Understanding MMS*.

www.mmswebsites.com
International list of retailers that sell MMS

4. Training Courses with Jim Humble

Jim Humble offers a number of training seminars each year, at present mainly in Costa Rica and Mexico. Courses are taught in English. The course programme cover all protocols, exercises in the practical use of MMS and how to produce it, and of course all the latest developments in the field.

Check Jim Humble's website (www.jimhumble.biz) for details of the

Further information on MMS

next course, or write (in English) to *mmsforhispaniola@gmail.com*. For information on the Puerto Vallarta Seminar in Mexico, contact *healthvallarta@gmail.com*.

For seminars in Costa Rica, write to *lukasjlouw@gmail.com*.

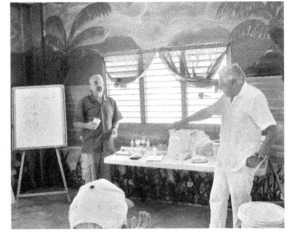

Due to the high volume of emails received on everything to do with MMS and the small number of staff dealing with them, it may be some time before you receive an answer. It is possible that email addresses or course locations may change.

If you do not receive an answer to your email, you will find all the latest information on Jim Humble's website (www.jimhumble.biz), as well as information on other seminar locations such as Argentina, Brazil, Bulgaria, the Dominican Republic, Ecuador and Peru (correct at time of printing). The seminar is also available on DVD.

Legal aspects

Approved for sterilising drinking-water in Germany

When taking MMS you are doing so on your own responsibility. The ingredients of MMS (sodium chlorite + activating acid) have only been approved in order to produce a chlorine dioxide solution to sterilise water. Since Jim Humble first made public the wonderful results he has had with MMS, numerous attempts have been made from various quarters to hinder his work. As a result of these developments, Jim Humble decided to establish a church for health and healing to protect those who produce, sell or take MMS from prosecution.

Protection from compulsory vaccination

He also wants to give people who live in states where vaccination is compulsory the option of protecting themselves from enforced vaccination. In the USA, for example, a child will be given more than 40 vaccines by the time they reach the age of 17. They are sometimes given forcibly, against the wishes of the parents or child.

It is difficult to predict how the legal situation will develop. Spain recently prohibited the sale of MMS for a short period, before allowing it again. In Germany, opportunities to buy MMS are limited at present (January 2015) since the authorities have demanded that a number of retailers stop selling the product.

Medication similar to MMS approved

In 2009, chlorine dioxide under the name 'Dioxychlor' was used as an infusion treatment at the Seegarten Klinik in Zurich, and the information provided stated that it could be used with the following indications:

flu, herpes I and II, hepatitis B, Epstein-Barr, cytomegaly, polio, toxoplasmosis and TB. Dioxychlor was also successfully used to treat virulent fungal infections such as candida albicans, mycoplasma, blood parasites, and pleomorphic bacteria, which mainly occur in cases of multiple allergies. Other areas of use include treatment after long-term use of antibiotics and the resulting harm, such as chronic fatigue syndrome (CFS, Epstein-Barr, HHV-6 virus). The successful implementation of Dioxychlor treatment in Europe and the USA has resulted in the expansion of the indication list to include other illnesses in addition to those mentioned above. These include gum infections, immune system weaknesses, cystic fibrosis, recurrent lung infections and bronchial pneumonia with recurrent infections.

Despite these successes, it is no longer listed as one of the treatments on offer. However, if you search for 'Dioxychlor' on the Seegarten Klinik website, you will find an information leaflet (in German) that provides a summary of important information regarding Dioxychlor. The leaflet states that Dioxychlor is neither toxic to cells nor are there any contra-indications known. It also states that Dioxychlor has been clinically used more than 50,000 times, including in Mayo Clinics.

You will find more information in chapter 8.7 'MMS in intravenous infusions'.

In the USA, the FDA has applied so much pressure that the company Green Life, which sold MMS, has decided to recall all the bottles of MMS it has ever sold. The companies that still sell MMS don't know for how much longer they will be able to do so.

This is despite the fact that there is no indication that MMS use in the recommended dosage has ever had a harmful effect. It is possible that MMS will not be available in future for legal reasons, at least not under that name. The authorities in the UK, Canada, France, the Netherlands, and Switzerland all advise against taking MMS because it can cause nausea and diarrhoea. If you live in a country that has forbidden the sale of MMS, you could try the following search terms: 'drinking-water steriliser', 'drinking-water purifier', '0.29% chlorine dioxide solution', or '22.5% sodium chlorite solution'. You now know how to use these substances if you decide to do so on your own responsibility. *No indications of harm resulting from MMS use*

Alternative search terms

But things may turn out differently and MMS could officially be approved for use as a medication. It is largely up to us.

If vaccinations no longer bring in large profits for pharmaceutical companies because no one wants to be vaccinated any more, and if the 'market' for antibiotics collapses because MMS works well as an antibiotic and comes, as far as we know, without side effects, then it might make financial sense for the pharmaceutical companies to go after a share of the MMS market – but probably not before the demand from patients makes it worth their while.

We have a responsibility in this area.

If you have had positive experiences with MMS and want MMS to continue to be available, I would urge you to become involved in the MMS campaign in whatever way you can, for example in relation to

17 • *Legal aspects*

your MP, administrative bodies, government authorities and the media.

You can also respond to defamatory reports in the media by writing letters, making phone calls or by commenting on the internet. In one instance in Germany, a number of people were infuriated by erroneous claims made on radio and TV programmes regarding the dangers of MMS. They left comments on www.br.de/nachrichten/gefaehrliche-schlankheitsmacher-internet-100.html stating that they, in contrast to the journalist's claims, had only ever had positive, curative effects from MMS. All these responses (there were over 60) were, tellingly, deleted within four days by the Bavarian broadcaster without comment, and the comment function was deactivated.

CENSOR-SHIP! Your involvement is vital

This incident has been documented with screenshots, see: https://kulturstudio.wordpress.com/tag/miracle-mineral-supplement/

It is also scandalous that the Red Cross is apparently not interested in MMS, despite the fact that a study on MMS was conducted under the leadership of the Red Cross in Uganda. As part of this clinical pilot study by the Red Cross, MMS was given to sick patients over the course of 4 days at a medical centre in Luuka in Uganda. Laboratory tests confirmed that no malaria was detectable in the blood of the patients within 24–48 hours of taking 18 drops of activated MMS, and that 100% of the malaria patients were clinically healthy after taking MMS.

Leo Koehof has produced a 20-minute documentary film (in German) on this topic, see: *www.youtube.com/watch?v=ZOO3U7PkXOw*; or alternatively visit www.daniel-peter-verlag.de and click on the video featuring the Red Cross.

This happened in December 2012. The Red Cross has still not taken any steps to make these facts known to the world or to use this cheap and simple measure to help cure the many people who are suffering and dying from malaria. Instead, they are demanding that the video be taken down from the internet!

Malaria could be cured but the Red Cross appears not to be interested. That should make us stop and think, and it reminds us of our own responsibilities. After all, you can always let the Red Cross know what you think by writing emails and letters, and in the way you choose to donate money.

Guidelines for healthy living

Regarding maintaining health, there is no such thing as universally valid rules that apply to everyone equally.

What I can tell you is in which areas of life you need to be particularly attentive if you want to maintain or recover your health. If some of this is familiar to you move on and begin reading again from whatever point catches your attention.

Awareness will help you find what really is good for your health. *Awareness*

That can be very different from one person to the next. Something that makes one person ill can be excellent for another. Take sport as an example. While one person might feel fine giving it their all, it can be very harmful for another person, especially if they demand more from their body than it can cope with. The important thing is to find the right balance – and this is true for everyone. If you are unsure what is good for your health and what is not, here are two simple questions to help you decide:

'Do I feel good while I am doing it?' and 'Do I feel good after doing it?'

If, for example, you are comfortable with jogging five miles and you feel relaxed and content afterwards, you can assume that running such distances is good for you. But if you are bracing yourself for a battle of will against your body because you want to take part in a marathon at any cost, even though your physical body is not suited to it and you begin to torment yourself, forcing yourself to train, no longer taking care of yourself because you are focused only on your goal, a goal you have forced upon yourself with an iron will …

When it no longer feels light and joyful the results will sooner or later become apparent. Not to mention what will happen if you pump unnatural stimulants such as anabolic steroids into your body.

Professional sportsmen and women often pay a high price for their careers. It is a different matter if you get so much joy from your sport that you are happy to do it, and feel good during and after a session.

It is good to exert yourself if you listen to your body when it tells you when it is time to stop before you overstrain yourself. This way even a marathon can be healthy. But what is 'health'?

Over the course of time, various people and institutions have tried to specify what that means and a new definition is postulated every 10 to 30 years. Everyone has a personal understanding of what it means to be healthy. There are people who are severely disabled but who feel healthy, while there are others who are 'normal' according to all the tests modern medicine has to offer but, despite that, they feel ill.

Health is so hard to define because it straddles so many different levels and we usually only pay attention to it when it is lost.

Overacidification Overacidification is one aspect that is still completely ignored by modern medicine – apart from holistically-oriented doctors and alternative practitioners. Overacidification of the tissue happens gradually; the human organism can compensate for the results for a long time without allowing illnesses to develop. But over the years, little by little, it leaves its mark, for example in biofilm and deposits. The result is restricted function and increased susceptibility to infections.

It is an accepted fact in the field of natural and experiential medicine that an overacidic body represents an ideal breeding ground for all kinds of diseases. Two hundred years ago, Samuel Hahnemann, the founder of homeopathy, pointed out in his fundamental work *Organon of the Healing Art* that obstacles to healing must be removed if health is to be restored.

Among such obstacles he included emotional upsets such as anger, fear, worry or melancholy, as well as overstimulation through an unnatural diet or an unhealthy lifestyle due to excesses of any kind.

Alongside excesses of food and stimulants such as sugar, alcohol, caffeine, cigarettes or drugs, this can include too much television, work or sport. Doctors have now even recognised addiction to mobile phones as a condition. No matter in what area of life – too much is too much. If the particular stress continues for too long, overacidification ensues. I therefore recommend adding less acid when activating MMS than is usually recommended (see chapter 6.2 'Acid–alkaline balance').

MMS leads to the oxidisation of pathogenic microbes and other harmful substances and therefore helps, in many cases, to cure diseases. But it is wise to take steps to change the long-term state of overacidification.

In my opinion that is the best preventative health measure you can take. There is much to gain from understanding that your body only sends signals of disease when you are well out of balance. Diseases do not just appear out of the blue. You have produced them yourself and have prepared the ground for them. Taking MMS or some other medication while leaving everything else in your life as it is does not represent a good long-term solution. It is necessary to combat the disease as well as to take time to establish a healthy lifestyle. I will explain and give examples of what you can do to avoid overacidification and to bring your body back to a state of health. Based on my knowledge of kinesiology I work with five bodies: the physical body, the electrical / emotional body, the mental body, the dream body and the soul body. Each one can become unbalanced, thereby causing a negative impact on your health. If that persists over a long period of time, illness manifests itself. Illnesses show that something is not right, sometimes in astoundingly simple ways. If, for example, you have 'had it up to here' (pointing towards your head / nose area) and are repressing this feeling, it is quite possible that you will develop a cold. Your body allows the rhinovirus to settle and spread – which it would not usually have done – because the physical body serves as an outlet. If your nose is literally full of mucus and you have noticed this condition, the idiom 'had it up to here' has found a physical expression. Once it has been sufficiently expressed it can, quite simply, disappear. We then discover to our relief that we become well again. In acute cases the matter is over. But if you are constantly angry and repress this feeling, chronic illness can develop. Since conventional medicine only treats symptoms on the physical level, it is impossible to bring about healing on a deeper level. Symptom-orientated medicine can only suppress symptoms of illness and in some cases you will have to remain on medications for the remainder of your life. True healing can only come about when the deeper emotional level is addressed.

Health-promoting lifestyle

The physical body as an outlet

If a patient becomes aware of and resolves long-fostered resentments in a session of kinesiology or psychotherapy, the body can cease to serve as an outlet, for example via joint and muscle pains, and the patient feels healthy again. A cure can only come about if you treat the body in which the disharmony is located. Treating just the physical body is of little use if the origin of the illness is not to be found there.

This is also true of MMS. If you keep falling ill, it is worth looking for the root cause. Based on my clinical experience, I would say that most illnesses in developed countries occur because of emotional imbalance.

During the course of our socialisation, we are usually not encouraged

Disease occurs as a result of emotional imbalance to deal openly with emotions within the family, at school, or in society more generally. As a result very few people have learned to be aware of their emotions and to act upon that awareness adequately, that is, in a way that promotes health. Pressures in the workplace have increased dramatically over the last few decades. While one section of society is overworked and becomes ill as a result, another section becomes ill because they cannot find work.

Thorough examination and case history The causes of illness can be complex and multilayered. To help the patient regain health in the long term, the doctor must take the case history and make a thorough examination, as is done in homeopathy. It is then necessary to consider how to begin treatment. You will be asked first of all for your opinion, so that the process can advance as swiftly and effectively as possible. Health can only return to the extent that you are willing to get to know yourself better, and to become aware of, to honour, and to express your emotions. This can happen quickly if you release old habits and disease-promoting attitudes that do you no good. This can be seen clearly in cases of acute illnesses. In chronic illness, the causes are often complex and multilayered. Healing takes time in such cases. Experience from the field of homeopathy shows that an illness that has lasted a year will require about a month to cure; illnesses that have lasted 25 years will require about 25 months. Patience and an inner resolve to play an active part and to take responsibility for your own health will help. And now we come to what you can do for your health.

18.1 LIVING CONSCIOUSLY: THOUGHTS AND EMOTIONS

Your thoughts primarily determine your well-being and therefore your health. That is true of people who have all their basic needs met, such as oxygen, water, food, clothing, and a roof over their heads.

If you are happy, you have a much greater chance of becoming or staying healthy compared to being unhappy, discontented, angry or resentful. Old and deeply entrenched emotions such as malice, hate, worry, guilt, jealousy or resentment are particularly likely to lead to illness.

The good news is that you, through your thoughts, produce and perpetuate these emotions yourself, but you can also resolve and release them. If you observe your thoughts, you will discover whether or not you treat yourself and others in a friendly and loving way. Try it. You will be surprised how many negative thoughts you have regarding yourself, others, and your living conditions, over the course of a day.

Thoughts produce emotions, emotions determine the words we use and the deeds we do – all of these together produce the state of our health.

What can you do when you notice that you are tormenting yourself with thoughts that do you no good?

There are a number of options available, depending on your level of perseverance.

1. You have realised that you no longer want to have a certain thought. Whenever the thought arises, decide to allow it to move on, don't worry about it, and think about something else.
   When you have practised that a few times and it is working, at some point the thought will no longer arise because you have deprived it of energy. This often works. Just try it. Be brave and good luck!
2. Perhaps method 1 did not work for you. Incidentally, that can happen although you may have used it successfully with other thoughts. But perhaps for this certain thought if just doesn't do the trick ...
   After all, you really are right, if the others were just not so mean ...
   If you really want to put an end to your suffering, I recommend you read *Loving What Is* by Byron Katie. By means of a short process, she makes it possible for you to change the thoughts that you nurture regarding your problem, and all in a beautifully simple way. But, of course, only if you want to do so.
   Take a simple example. You feel that your partner should give you more care and attention. At the moment he is not giving you as much loving attention as you would like because he is busy with other things (sports club, the community, politics ...). Every time he leaves the house in the evenings, you think 'My partner should give me more loving attention', and you suffer. If, for example, you could think: 'It is great that he has a fulfilling activity so that I have time for myself every now and again, or time to learn to play a musical instrument', or something to that effect, then you would feel good even though the external circumstance has not changed at all.
   Thoughts are free. This means that you can always choose what you want to think. Below is Byron Katie's process.
   You ask yourself four questions, there is a turnaround, and a conclusion. 'Turnaround' means that you first write down the exact opposite of your first statement; then change the name of the persons who

Simple process to release negative thoughts and feelings by Byron Katie – one example

irritate you to 'I' or 'my thoughts'; and thirdly change the people involved, which also leads to a kind of turnaround of the first statement. This will all become much clearer with an example:

> Assume that you are suffering because your partner is not giving you as much loving care and attention as you would like. Formulate a statement that expresses this.
>
> *Statement:* My partner should give me more loving care and attention.
> *First question:* Is that really true?
> *Answer:* Yes. If you answer 'no', continue with question 2. If not, answer the following supplementary question.
> *Supplementary question:* Can I say with 100% certainty that that is absolutely true?
> *Answer:* Perhaps.
>
> *Second question:* How do I feel when I have this thought?
> *Answer:* Sad, angry, worthless.
>
> *Third question:* How would I feel if I did not have to have this thought?
> *Answer:* Happy, content, precious, valued.

Now the fact is that the woman in our example, like everyone else, is free to choose her thoughts. She does not have to hold on to this thought. She can decide to hold on to it, and perhaps to old history in the form of memories, until she feels really bad, or she can release it because she wants to feel happy, content, precious and valued.

> *Fourth question:* Is there a good reason why you should hold on to this thought?
>
> 'Good reason' here means a rational reason; is it rational to keep the thought, in the sense that you feel good with the thought? This is, after all, the purpose of the exercise. In this process, there is usually never a good reason for writing 'yes' here because if you did not suffer as a result of the thought you would not have begun the exercise in the first place.

Answer: No, there is no good reason to hold on to this thought. If you were able to wrestle your way through to this conclusion then you have already taken a big step forward.

The first turnaround – the exact opposite

'My partner should give me more loving care and attention' is turned around to: 'My partner should not give me more loving care and attention.' That sounds harsh. If you just screamed: 'No, but he should!' then start the exercise again from the beginning. After all, you want to let go of the thought. At this point you are testing yourself to see whether or not you have let go of it. If you are still raging inside it means that you are not there yet. The only thing that will help is for you to look inside yourself and ask 'What do I really want?'

The fact is that your partner is not giving you the loving care and attention that you want at the moment. Your resistance to that does nothing to change the situation. All that happens is that you are banging your head against a wall and are getting a bloody nose for the hundredth time. If you can accept that your partner should not give you more loving attention when he is not doing so, then you have won.

This does not mean that he generally should not be giving you more attention. The turnaround statement refers to that moment in which he is not doing so and you feel he should be giving you more attention. After all, he is not doing that at the moment anyway. As you have seen above, you can put an end to your suffering if you accept that. If you tell yourself: 'Oh, if he's not doing that right now, then he shouldn't do it' – then you are interrupting your cycle of negative thoughts. You can, of course, talk to your partner irrespective of this process but that is not the focus here. What we are doing here is accepting something that is happening, something you cannot change. But you can change your attitude. That is in your hands.

Second turnaround

Replace the person or institution that is irritating you with 'I' or 'my thoughts'.

'My partner should give me more loving care and attention' becomes 'I should give myself more loving care and attention', or 'My thoughts should give me more loving care and attention.'

It is especially rewarding to take some time over this stage. Could it be that you do not give yourself enough loving care and attention?

To be honest, that is very likely. If we gave ourselves enough loving care and attention, we would not be so dependent on receiving it from others. But once you have arrived at the realisation that you (or your thoughts) need to give yourself more loving care and attention, you hold all the aces.

If you feel you should do that, and you want to do that, who is going to stop you from doing it? No one can do that except you. If you are now thinking something like 'Yes, but I can't, my family needs me', continue by saying 'My family should not make such demands of me.' Let us first finish this exercise.

Third turnaround

'My partner should give me more loving care and attention' becomes 'I should give my partner more loving care and attention.' Ask yourself again: 'Could that also be true?' From his perspective, perhaps he needs more loving care and attention in the sense that you develop an understanding for the reasons behind the way he behaves.

To conclude

To make absolutely sure that you really are well prepared for the next time whatever irritates you happens, write out the following:
I am ready once again to experience what I previously did not want – in this case that my partner does not show me more loving care and attention.
If you have come this far and are able to look at the situation with a peaceful heart, your suffering concerning this matter will be at an end.

Regardless of whether or not your partner pays more or less attention to you, you can now be happy and content, and feel precious and protected because you have chosen that.

The funny thing is that it is likely that your partner, over the next weeks or months, will probably give you more loving care and attention because he does not want to miss the pleasure of being around you and your happy and contented aura.

You can use this model to process and release all the resentments and pains for which you hold someone else responsible. You can use

Katie Byron's brilliant suggestion as a kind of psychotherapeutic self-treatment.

I like working with this because I like simple, effective methods. You will find further examples, detailed explanations, and much more in Byron Katie, *Loving What Is* (Rider, 2002).

3. If you do not get any results from this either, it is likely that certain subconscious patterns, beliefs and programming are at the root of your problems. I assume that you have made a genuine attempt at the previous exercises. In such cases, kinesiology sessions are enormously helpful. Some students of mine who themselves work as therapists are surprised again and again at how much can be achieved with so little effort. Through the use of simple muscle testing, kinesiology allows you to communicate with your subconscious. It is astonishing how your muscles can give precise information regarding what is good for you and what is not, when and why a trauma, problem or stress arose, together with information such as which exercises you need to perform, or what information you need to have in order to resolve a problem. You cannot ask every question that is on your mind because your inner wisdom decides whether now is the correct time to deal with a particular topic or not. Another issue might need to be resolved first, for example you may not have the necessary stability to process a certain problem. A number of sessions may be necessary in order to deal with a problem in its entirety. But much more is possible than most people imagine before they have tried it out for themselves. Below is an example of how a kinesiology treatment might proceed.

Kinesiology

> A 10-year-old girl comes for a treatment for atopic dermatitis. She has had sensitive skin ever since she was an infant. Since going to high school her skin has been breaking out in an itchy rash which makes her scratch, causing further inflammation. It has been so bad recently that she has had to take a number of antibiotics and cortisone creams to heal the open wounds. The skin is the organ that establishes the border between us and the outside world. In the symbolism of the language of the organs, a skin eruption can be translated as 'You are pushing at my boundaries, leave me in peace.'
> By asking targeted questions and carrying out the kinesiology arm tests, it became apparent that the girl was finding it hard to keep

Example of a treatment session based on the principles of kinesiology up with the work at high school and felt under constant pressure because she was ambitious and wanted to score good marks. In the first session she succeeded in resolving the stress resulting from her own expectations and the expectations of others. A test was done to find the homeopathic remedy that would be ideally suited to her at that time. Over nine weeks, her skin improved so much that she no longer needed to use medical creams at all. The skin is still dry and red in patches but the itching has almost completely gone and the skin had not opened in six weeks. Using the arm test, we ask whether it would be good to continue to resolve stress issues. The arms say 'yes' so we searched for further stress factors and discover that she finds it distressing that her class is so large and restive. Such issues can be resolved with kinesiology. This does not mean that she is now happy regarding the constant unrest but she does not suffer so much that it makes her ill. She finds it easier to concentrate even if the class is unsettled from time to time. As a result, she can take in more at school and requires less time with her homework. This means she has more time for herself, which, in turn, leads to a more balanced emotional state. Since she no longer puts herself under so much pressure with regard to her marks, she is relaxed when approaching tests. When she comes to the third consultation after a further three months, her skin is almost free of symptoms. The girl now enjoys going to school, has achieved some Bs in tests (she previously gained Cs and Ds) and currently has no skin abnormalities. We ask the arms again. No more issues need to be resolved at present. So I discharge the girl and tell her to get in touch if the condition of her skin deteriorates, or if she experiences any other symptoms.

That was an example of a typical treatment. It is rare to solve the whole problem in one session. In persistent cases stress-releasing sessions may be required every two to four months for a number of years to cure or alleviate the symptoms. I cannot promise in advance that the illness will be cured, or if it is cured, when that will happen. However, based on my experience, I can say that the majority of patients are very satisfied with the results. Whether or not a recovery takes place depends largely on the patient. The patient can become well to the extent that they are ready to release whatever is making them ill. Kinesiology, with its specialised technique, can play a helpful supporting role in that process. Generally speaking, children regain their health more quickly than adults, and acute illnesses are easier to treat than chronic illnesses. The skin usually only heals when everything inside the body is in harmony. With kinesiology we have the wonderful possibility of approaching the problem on an individual basis, to test which stress factors, which are usually subconscious, lie at the root of the symptoms and to resolve these as far as that is possible.

There are many kinesiology exercises which help to balance the muscles, harmonise autonomic functions, improve lymph flow, improve co-operation between the hemispheres of the brain, and much more. These exercises can be done in groups or on your own. They help to balance an existing problem for a while but you must repeat the exercise every now and again because the effect fades. A kinesiology session uses these exercises to deal with stress but goes much deeper. In the session, the root cause of the stress is identified and resolved. I like to compare it to weeding out dandelion roots: if you have pulled out the whole root then it cannot grow back. By doing this, situations that had previously caused an enormous amount of stress are now perceived as being far less strenuous. The mind is no longer compromised by old fears and beliefs, at least as far as the special topics successfully treated in kinesiology sessions are concerned. If you want to know more about this field, I recommend *Tools of the Trade* by Gordon Stokes and Daniel Whiteside (VAK Verlag, 2011), ISBN 978-3-924077-16-9, which offers a clear introduction to the possibilities offered by kinesiology. *Recommended reading*

Kinesiology testing can be used to find the optimal remedy. In my practice, that is usually homeopathic remedies or flower essences. The correct homeopathic remedy at the correct potency – the so-called simile – works quickly and effectively, especially in acute illnesses.

I have not compiled statistics but I believe I can honestly say that, in my practice over the last 20 years, I have only had to prescribe antibiotics once every few years or so. I sometimes test and find that another treatment should take priority, such as osteopathy, music therapy, acupuncture, SOMA therapy, physiotherapy, massage, energy essence medicines, ayurvedic medicine, Erich Körbler's healing symbols, healing crystals, and many other treatment forms.

In such cases it is necessary to use that treatment first, before asking whether or not a homeopathic remedy is necessary. Or it can be good to combine both, or a number of other treatments.

Example Take a person with chronic back pain for example. After taking a case history, the kinesiology test might reveal the following.
1. The patient has been dehydrated for too long. They need to drink 2.5 litres of water every day.
2. The belief 'I have to do everything myself' prevents the patient from relaxing. The kinesiology test uncovers this unconscious belief, which is resolved through kinesiology exercises.

The healing exercises mentioned originate from the old wisdom of the Chinese, Indian and Egyptian cultures, as well as from the discoveries of modern brain research and psychotherapy. These are combined with the experience gathered by kinesiologists over the last 60 years while using these methods, and with much that has been developed by kinesiologists themselves. But let us return to the example.

Example continued In the case of the man with chronic back problems, I test and discover that:
3. he should take the homeopathic remedy Bryonia at the LM 18 potency twice a day for five weeks.

Dear readers, please do not go away and take Bryonia, and certainly not twice a day for five weeks. The chances that this is the correct treatment for you are less than one in a thousand. Taking the wrong remedy for such a long time can lead to you 'proving' the remedy. This means that the remedy shows you which symptoms it can cure. And that means that you suffer from the exact symptoms of disease that Bryonia LM 18 can produce. In some cases it can take a while for these to subside.

Homeopathic remedies Homeopathic remedies are powerful and very effective medicines when expertly prescribed. Higher potencies should therefore be used with due caution, that is, do not use them at all if you are not well versed in homeopathy. A completely different medicine or treatment may be better suited in your case.

Our back pain patient has had the Bryonia remedy specially tested for him and his condition. So I can assume that it will be the best course of treatment for him. The tests also reveal that osteopathic treatment would be a good supportive therapy. In his case this is not absolutely necessary but it will help him to feel better more quickly. It can take a while before all the twisted muscular structures, fascia, tendons, discs and joints are back where they belong, depending on how long they have been out of place. Everything moves much faster with a little energetic and mechanical coaxing. The good news is that the back remains pain-free as long as there is no internal stress to cause the muscles to contract again. However, if there are further sources of stress to resolve, osteopathic treatment alone will not be enough. That is why a holistic course of treatment that addresses both internal and external, both mental and physical factors, is so beneficial.

Our patient is sent home with a prescription for Bryonia LM 18 (twice a day), instructed to drink 2.5 litres of water daily, and advised to make an appointment with an osteopath. When he returns to the clinic in eight weeks he will probably feel much better. In my experience, he will need to come three times a year for the next four years. After that he feels well and I only hear from him every now and again, that is, a year or two may pass without an appointment. He has learned to look after himself, to drink plenty of water, not to take on more than is good for him, and to seek help when he needs it, for example a session of osteopathy or kinesiology. In this way he can manage very well. With chronic problems I would recommend psychotherapy. It is much better than its reputation would have you believe. I have only heard of a few patients who regret undergoing psychotherapy, especially in the areas of depth-oriented psychotherapy, behaviour therapy, and body-oriented therapies. It would actually do most people good to spend 30 to 50 hours engaging with themselves and their emotions with the benefit of professional counselling.

Psychotherapy is sadly still considered taboo by many people. However, the main purpose of such a treatment is not to cure serious mental illnesses such as schizophrenia or severe depression; that is often not possible using only psychotherapy. The main purpose is to resolve neuroses, traumas, or behavioural disorders, after which life can become significantly more pleasant. Even if it is uncomfortable to be told this, it is likely that you too have a small neurosis, just as I do, and your neighbour, the baker, and your boss. It is actually quite difficult to find someone who does not. There is a good possibility that you would gain insights through psychotherapy which would be of benefit to you throughout your life.

Psychotherapy

A study was carried out at the psychology department of Leipzig University on patients who wanted to undergo an operation on their intervertebral discs because of back pain. The researchers were able to assess from a questionnaire filled in by the patients beforehand which patients would later regard the operation a success because they had less pain, which patients would be helped by psychotherapy, and which patients would see no improvement, neither from the operation nor from psychotherapy. The percentages predicted matched the actual results almost exactly. Since the statistics on the success rate of operations on intervertebral discs are not particularly impressive in terms of pain relief, this study is of particular interest to me because it shows:

1. that psychotherapy can, in many cases, help the operation to be successful
2. that so much depends on the patient. If they are unwilling, either subconsciously or otherwise, no cure will come about. Thankfully that also works the other way around. If they can let go of what is making them ill, and if their soul wants to become well, the patient can heal any illness, no matter what the diagnosis.

Read examples of this in *Getting Well Again* by O. Carl Simonton, who worked with patients for whom all treatment options were exhausted. However, this requires you to be actively engaged and to take responsibility for your own health.

The first stage is to work on emotional aspects by resolving old anger and resentments – and that brings us back full circle to the benefits of kinesiology and psychotherapy.

18.2 LIVING CONSCIOUSLY: THE PHYSICAL BODY

The human body is delighted if any attention whatsoever is paid to it without it first having to cry for attention by giving pain signals.

If you do not know how to do that, simply assume that your body has both intelligence and feelings. Every second, millions of finely regulated processes take place in just a single cell. The micro reflects the macro.

Using a sufficiently powerful microscope, it would be possible to see that there is at least as much going on in a single cell in your body as there is in a large city. Power plants producing energy, transport vehicles, waste incineration plants, the list goes on. Everything is working together with efficiency and precision. There exist wonderful images of this by the photographer Lennart Nilsson. If you want to acquire a deeper understanding of this area and have the time to study the foundations of physiology, I recommend the *Color Atlas of Physiology* by Stefan Silbernagl and Agamemnon Despopoulos (Thieme) ISBN 978–3135450063.

You can feel safe in the knowledge that your body is wonderfully equipped; it knows what is good for you and how to ensure survival better than your conscious mind does. So listen to it.

It signals tiredness when it needs sleep.

It signals thirst when it needs water.

It signals hunger when it needs food.

More importantly, it signals when it has had enough, for example when it is full, overstrained or simply in need of a rest.

Your physical body needs sufficient oxygen, water and salt, as well as loving care and attention, just as much as it needs sufficient food. It needs movement and rest / sleep, and it needs clothing and shelter because there are only a few areas on this planet with climates that allow humans to live fully exposed to the elements.

I have compiled a checklist of areas in which we need to pay attention to our bodies. If you take the time to answer the questions, you will see for yourself how you can take better care of yourself.

18.3 PHYSICAL HEALTH CHECKLIST

- Am I getting enough fresh air?   *Checklist*
- Am I drinking enough water? An average-sized adult needs about 2.5 litres of water per day.
  Is the water I drink pure and of good quality?
- Do I eat what is good for me in the correct amounts? Do I take my time to choose and prepare my food?
- How do I use my energy? Do I have enough rest, sleep and leisure time? Do I have enough movement?
- Do I choose my hygiene products, clothes and shoes with care?
- Have I taken measures to ensure that I can sleep without being disturbed?
  Have I designed my home and workplace so that I feel good there?
- Do I have a comprehensive knowledge of vaccinations?

18.3.1 Living consciously: fresh air

Humans need oxygen for survival more than we need anything else. We should be concerned with keeping the air we breathe as clean as possible and avoid everything that pollutes it, not only for ourselves as individuals but also for the survival of our species. Forests are particularly important because they clean the air by taking in carbon dioxide and turning it into oxygen.

What each of us does counts in this regard. The situation will not improve by waiting. What can you do? For every tree you fell, plant two new ones. Tell your friends, colleagues and the politicians representing you that protecting the climate is your first priority because humans cannot live on this earth without sufficient oxygen.

And what can you do for your own health? Take every opportunity to go out into the open air. Do some errands on foot or on your bike every now and again. Take the stairs instead of the lift. If you want more fresh air you will find a number of small, unspectacular opportunities during the day when you can get some fresh air. And when you notice that that produces a good feeling in your body and is achieved without much effort, you will want to do it again at the next opportunity.

18.3.2 Living consciously: water and salt

Water is the second most important element that humans need. The one need that is more immediate is the air we breathe. Water is the foundation of life. It stores information and passes it on. Live water supplies us with regulative energy and it must be available within and outside human cells in sufficient quantity to allow metabolic processes to occur. Lack of water stresses the body. The organism can no longer adequately dispose of its waste products and can only keep other processes going in a limited way. A person will slowly die after about ten days without water. A 40-day fast, in contrast, can be beneficial for a human, assuming they take in plenty of water and salt.

Reading suggestion   You will find interesting facts regarding water in *Water and Salt: The Essence of Life* by Dr Barbara Hendel and Peter Ferreira. They explain how the water in Germany contains 300 pesticides and fungicides, how the structure of tap water is destroyed by the pressure in the water pipes and no longer has the structure of live spring water, and how carbonated or ozonised mineral waters are 'dead' and no longer have health-giving properties.

I have seen a number of patients in my practice who have not needed any medication. They only needed an adequate quantity of water to become well again. Natural, live spring water is certainly the best. But if you cannot obtain that, it helps to just revitalise your tap water with a handful of quartz, amethyst and rose quartz. Do this by placing the stones in a jug, pour water onto them and leave that to stand for a few hours before you drink it. If your water is heavily chlorinated, it is advisable to filter it beforehand: first filter, then revitalise. If in doubt, it is certainly better to drink any water than not to drink anything because you are worried you don't have the perfect water. You will find out how much is right for you after observing your feelings of thirst for a few weeks. I recommend 2 to 2.5 litres of water for an average-sized adult. You can adapt this to your body size. If you multiply your weight in kg by 30ml you will find your ideal amount of water, for example 70kg: 70 x 30ml = 2100ml = 2.1 litres. *Your need for water*

If you have been drinking significantly less than this for many years and you are chronically ill, your daily requirement may be as high as 3–4 litres. If you start with 2.5 litres and increase by 100ml per week, you will find out how much water your body really needs. If you generally dislike drinking-water, it would be a good idea to have a kinesiology session to resolve that because it will not be easy to become well again without drinking an adequate amount of water.

Salt is needed to regulate water levels in the body. These days salt is industrially 'cleaned', which means that minerals such as potassium, calcium, magnesium, and many trace elements that are usually present in small quantities in ancient rock salt, are synthetically removed during the refining process. What remains is pure sodium chloride. In most cases, that is then iodised. A huge range of preservatives are often added, including calcium carbonate, magnesium carbonate, E535, E536, E540, E550, E551, E552, E553b, E570, E572, and aluminium hydroxide, which improves the free-flowing quality and granulation. Aluminium is suspected of causing Alzheimer's disease. Cooking salt produced in this way is highly aggressive and not suitable for human consumption in the long term. In addition, most people use too much salt, resulting in the body having to use valuable minerals and cell water to eliminate the excess cooking salt. I salt my food rather sparingly because of this and I only use ancient rock salt, preferably Himalayan salt. Ancient rock salt *Preservatives* still contains all the necessary minerals and trace elements because it has not been refined. In theory, sea salt would be just as suitable but I prefer rock salt because the seas are so polluted in many areas. You can easily find Himalayan salt in most organic and health food shops or on the internet and it will probably make a noticeable difference to your health without much effort on your part.

Drinking enough liquids may be somewhat harder. If you don't like water, mix in some juice or drink rooibos tea, but if you do so you should drink higher quantities because the physical body uses water to process the additional substances. So if you want to drink 3 litres of water and you have drunk 0.5 litres of apple juice mixed with water, consider that as about 0.3 litres. Strictly speaking, it depends how much apple juice you added. When mixed in a 1:1 ratio, you have only covered 250ml of your daily requirement. When drinking rooibos tea, I calculate one-third of the quantity of tea towards the total daily requirement. It does not hinge on every last 100ml – the important thing is that you are drinking plenty of water. Nobody can do that for you.

Once you have understood how important and wonderful water is for your well-being, you may find it easier to drink all the water you need. The following books contain very interesting information on the topic of water and salt:

Reading suggestions

Dr Barbara Hendel and Peter Ferreira, *Water and Salt: The Essence of Life* (Natural Resources, 2003), ISBN 978-0974451510

F. Batmanghelidj M.D., *Your Body's Many Cries for Water* (Global Health), ISBN 978-0970245885

Dr Masaru Emoto, *The Hidden Messages in Water* (Pocket Books; 2005), ISBN 978-1416522195

18.3.3 Living consciously: food

There are a few things to remember if you hope to acquire energy and power from the food you eat.

Only buy food that deserves to be called 'food'. Top quality food can be recognised from the fact that it can 'go off'. The reason you can leave refined white sugar or flour for a few years without it going bad is because it no longer really deserves to be called food. Nutritional components that contain live energy can rot, become mouldy or decay in some way – that is why they are removed. Most convenience products consist of foods processed in this way so that they can be preserved for months. That is very practical but has huge drawbacks. Calories can be preserved; vitamins do not fare so well. More than anything, however, it is the biophoton content and the structure of the food that is lost in many industrial food production processes – the food is largely without nutritional value as a result. You would not know where to start if the numbers on your bank account were randomly cobbled together in any old way. The meaning of your statement would be radically changed, in fact, the statement would be completely useless.

In just the same way, a whole grain, an apple, or any other real food, is more than the sum of its parts. Imagine that you need a specialist to do a certain job for you. Biochemically speaking, a living specialist is hardly distinguishable from one that has just died. Both are made up of exactly the same building blocks. But what was it that you wanted from the specialist? He can no longer give you any information. It is of no use to you if scientists in the field of chemistry, biochemistry and mechanics assure you that everything is in order regarding the specialist.

Experiments show that we humans should not interfere. We cannot know what damage will result because we do not always know what we are doing. The human body absorbs more calcium from one single carrot than it does from a calcium tablet, not because there is more calcium in it but because the body cannot transfer the calcium into the cells without the auxiliary substances that belong with it. These are not provided in the calcium tablet.

Pasteurisation, for example, destroys the information contained in milk. That makes no difference biochemically speaking, but it interferes with the living structure of the milk. That has led to a situation where children who drink the most pasteurised milk now have the worst teeth.

Consuming pasteurised milk has an even more devastating effect on calves. One calf died within three weeks after being exclusively fed pasteurised milk from its mother cow.

Why? The vitality of the milk is destroyed and the milk can no longer impart life to the calf.

This is exactly what food is for. Obviously, ultra-high-temperature processing reduces the quality of milk even further.

What I find to be the worst habit for health, however, is the deplorable custom of preparing food in a microwave oven. I would rather not eat than have food from the microwave. Food is changed so drastically when microwaved that cats that were kept in a room with artificial light and fed exclusively with microwaved food (even though they could freely choose from a range of food) died within a month. This was the result of a study carried out in England, cited in *Water and Salt: The Essence of Life* by Dr Barbara Hendel and the biophysicist Peter Ferreira (Natural Resources, 2003) ISBN 978-0974451510.

Reading suggestion

The cats died of malnutrition even though they had completely over-indulged. The molecular composition of the food is changed by the microwave radiation to such an extent that no resonant form of energy was measurable and even the chemistry of the substances had changed.

I ask myself why should humans be able to cope with this. It does not seem to me that we can. I suspect that microwaved food is one of the causes of metabolic dysfunction and obesity.

The true value of a specific food goes well beyond its calorie, vitamin, trace element and mineral content. Its value is determined by the quantity of light information that is transmitted to the person eating it. This light is needed for intercellular communication, among other things, as proven by Professor Fritz-Albert Popp. The light stored in the food is absorbed by the human body. The light-quanta (photons), which he calls biophotons, enable a kind of light-signal radio communication both within and between cells.

Eating high quality food improves the body's self-regulation; poor quality nutrition leads to chaos. If you want your body to be 'in order', there is little sense in filling it up with foods that lead to disorder, in extreme cases even leading to death. What it needs in order to be healthy is a pure, regulative, light-filled diet. It is your responsibility to ensure that it gets that. A week fasting with ancient salt solution and live water could be of more benefit than much of what you have previously tried. If you have never fasted before, it is advisable to read up on it or to seek advice from a doctor who has experience of fasting.

Recommended reading

Books such as Hellmut Lützner's *Successful Fasting: The Easy Way to Cleanse your Body of its Poisons* (Thorsons, 1990) ISBN 978-0722521304, provide the necessary instructions. The F. X. Mayr diet can help to cleanse a body in a state of imbalance. However, when you are getting started, what you eat from day to day is far more important than a good fasting regimen. The reason for this is that you need light energy every single day. Professor Fritz-Albert Popp has succeeded in developing a device that detects and measures the quantity of biophotons in food. It can distinguish between free-range eggs and eggs from battery farms – it is not difficult to guess which contain more light energy. Organic lettuce also leaves conventionally grown lettuce far behind in terms of the quantity of light it contains. At present, these biophoton measuring devices are not available to end users – they cost about 80,000 euros. But Professor Popp and his team at the Institute for Biophysics in Neuss, in collaboration with an American scientist, hope to develop a handy device suitable for day-to-day shopping at a price of about 100 euros.

Biophoton measuring device

That is a promising prospect because we will then be able to distinguish between light-filled and light-depleted foods, even if intuition and instinct are no longer equal to the task.

The way we bake bread these days has a disastrous effect for the same reasons. Flour is stored in stocks of bread mixes which keep for months and which are used little by little. In former times, freshly-milled flour would usually be baked within three days, often on the same day, thereby preserving all the nutrients. There are still some bakers who bake freshly-milled flour, especially organic bakers. If you make it known that you prefer to buy bread made with freshly-milled flour, more bakers would surely consider doing so.

Bake freshly-milled flour on the same day

Food does not become healthier when it is subjected to unnatural methods such as ultra-high-temperature processing or the addition of preservatives, acidifiers, artificial flavourings, flavour enhancers and colourings. There are usually limits to how much additives foods may contain, limits that are considered by the authorities to be safe. But no one knows what the effects of accumulation in the body are in the long term. Human cells have had time to become familiar with grains, fruit etc. since the beginnings of humanity. All the artificially created substances invented over the last few decades by humans are comparatively new. Based on what we are now witnessing, it is not doing us any good. Almost all the so-called diseases of civilisation can be traced back in large part to unhealthy diets.

So eat as natural a diet as possible: that means organic – or do you *want* to consume harmful substances?

Wholemeal foods and five handfuls of fruit and vegetables a day are the cornerstones of a healthy diet.

Motto

Studies Studies show that vegetarians live healthier and longer lives than meat-eaters. The largest study ever made was published in the *British Medical Journal* in 1994. Eleven thousand people from the same social strata and with largely similar lifestyles were surveyed. The study showed that vegetarians had higher values in almost all the health parameters studied in comparison to meat-eaters. The mortality rate was 20% lower among vegetarians, and the cancer mortality rate was 40% lower. Discover more about vegetarianism on the UK Vegetarian Society's website: www.vegsoc.org

Information You will provide yourself with an adequate level of vitamins, minerals and protein if you combine fruit and vegetables sensibly with whole grains, legumes, nuts and seeds. If you eat dairy products and eggs every now and again you will not suffer any deficiencies because humans need essential amino acids more than anything, not meat. Amino acids are found in plants. For a comprehensive list of reading recommendations on the theme of vegetarian diets, see the Vegetarian Society's website:
www.vegsoc.org

If you decide to eat meat nevertheless, it is advisable to keep an eye out for quality. I am not referring to contaminated meat here. The questions to consider are: how and where an animal has lived, was it allowed to roam happily or was it intensively farmed under torturous conditions, and what was it fed on. Intensive farming often makes animals ill, which means that enormous amounts of pharmaceutical medicines are required, including antibiotics, hormones, tranquilisers and other psychoactive drugs. Humans then consume the residues left in the meat. Poisons from the feed can also accumulate in meat and dairy products. Animals are still fed so-called concentrated feeds that contain carcasses and bone meal. For herbivores such as cattle, that can have dire consequences.

Motto Above all: enjoy your food, take your time when eating, and only eat until you are satisfied, not overfull.

In the long term, overeating can be unhealthy. To guarantee that you digest your food completely, it is best to **eat three meals a day** and to **leave an interval of 4 to 6 hours between meals** and **avoid eating after 9 p.m.**

Living consciously: food

That is true for most people in northern countries, with few exceptions. It is likely to be different in southern countries. Where customs have endured for centuries it means that our predecessors have eaten in that way for generations. That leaves genetic traces and has an effect on how and when we are able to digest or tolerate different kinds of foods well.

Incidentally, freshly-prepared fruit and vegetables are not only rich in natural vitamins but are also cheaper than ready meals. And you are helping the climate when you refrain from consuming meat. The total CO_2 emissions of the cattle industry are greater than that of all means of transport worldwide including cars and aeroplanes.
(Source: www.vebu.de/umwelt/probleme-der-viehwirtschaft/608)

To make matters worse, large expanses of forests are cleared in order to grow animal feed. One hectare of land can feed between 10 and 22 people when it is used to grow potatoes, soya or vegetables. When the same hectare is used for cattle farming only one person can live on it. That means that if the demand for meat were lower, more agricultural land would be available to feed people. So there could be enough food for everyone on this planet. I find it an ironic paradox that one part of humanity is becoming ill because of lack of food, while another part is endangering its health through overeating and excessive meat consumption.

If you do not grow fruit and vegetables in your own garden and are keen to buy quality food, look out for the organic logo. The term 'organic' is, in the context of organic farming, a protected term under EU law, as is 'produce of organic agriculture' and 'certified organic'.

Information

In accordance with this, foods labelled with the German organic seal must fulfil the following conditions.
They:
- cannot have been exposed to ionising radiation as a means of preservation
- cannot have been produced using genetic modification
- cannot have been produced using synthetic pesticides
- cannot have been produced using easily soluble mineral fertilizers
- may, however, contain up to 5% conventionally produced components – but this is limited to raw materials listed in appendix IV of the regulations.

Further information from the EU organic regulations:
- There are strict limits on the use of additives and auxiliary ingredients in processed products (Appendix IV a and b) – taste enhancers, artificial flavourings and colourings, and emulsifiers are not allowed.
- The import of raw ingredients and products from third countries is regulated and subject to rigorous batch-related testing.
- The use of pesticides is forbidden.

The following are mandatory:
- multiannual crop rotation
- species-appropriate husbandry
- animals fed using only organically produced feeds without added antibiotics or growth enhancers.

Under certain exceptional conditions, a GMO percentage above the threshold of 0.9% may be used in organic production if no feed completely free of genetically modified ingredients can be bought on the market at the time the farmer has to buy feed.
(Source: http://de.wikipedia.org/wiki/Bio-Siegel)

Information

Food production associations make even stricter demands.
- Bioland (Germany) demands circulatory organic-biological farming without artificial fertilizers, pesticides, or additives.
- Demeter (Biodynamic Association) guarantees biodynamic-organic circulatory agriculture according to anthroposophic principles without artificial fertilizers, pesticides, or additives.
- The Marine Stewardship Council's label may only be used on fish caught from sustainable sources.
- Naturland certifies textiles, clothing and cosmetics, in addition to food.
- Ecovin certifies organic wines, juices, grape wine and sparkling wines.

These days, because of the huge demand for organic produce, there are many different organic certification labels for various products. If you want to know exactly what quality standards a certain organic label represents, you can find more information online.

http://www.aboutorganics.co.uk/a-guide-to-organic-food-accreditation.html (English)
http://www.sacert.org/standards (English)
http://www.biobay.de/content/115-bio-siegel (German)

The website of the 'BUND für Umwelt und Naturschutz in Deutschland' [Friends of the Earth Germany] (www.bund.net) offers a good overview of common organic certification labels with ratings ranging from 'highly recommended' to 'not recommended'. If you search for 'Biosiegel' on the main page you can reach a page where you only need to click on the summary to be able to read the recommendation. The following associations have received the highest recommendation: Biokreis, Bioland, Biopark, Demeter, Ecoland, Ecovin, Gaea and Naturland. You will find further information on the websites of the respective associations, some of which are also available in English. The minimum standards required in order to hold the EU's organic label is also judged to be commendable. Take care when you see terms such as 'natural' or 'naturally produced': this does not mean that the product is organic. It is designed to appeal to and deceive shoppers who want to buy healthy products.

It is worth knowing what the requirements of certain certification labels are. Then decide for yourself whether or not you want to consume a product that fulfils these criteria. The foods on offer in organic stores usually originate from producers who were 'highly recommended' by the BUND. You can assume that all the produce sold at farm shops are either from that farm itself or fulfils the farm's own quality standards or is labelled with additional information. If you are unsure, it is never a bad idea to ask.

High quality food is naturally full of flavour. Once you allow yourself to enjoy the pleasure of organic food you will never want to go back to your old eating habits. Professor Fritz-Albert Popp writes in his book *Die Botschaft der Nahrung* [The Message of Food] (Zweitausendeins, 2005) ISBN 978-3861503194 (the book is not available in an English translation), that it has been proven that organically grown plants contain far more biophotons than conventionally grown plants. So not only are they more enjoyable, they also provide you with more energy. When the human body has had enough food, nutrients and biophotons, it feels full and satisfied. If you only consume 'empty' foods that contain hardly any life force, you will never really feel full, and you will continue to feel an urge to eat or will feel hungry again soon after eating. As a result,

Reading suggestion

18 • *Guidelines for healthy living*

you eat too much. In the long term that is more expensive than a nutrient-rich diet of organic fruit, vegetables and whole grains.

Food can taste good, be healthy, and provide good value: try it!

It is interesting to experiment with fresh herbs and spices. It is worth learning about these not only in order to add taste but also because they have medicinal properties. In Asian medical traditions food is considered a medicine. Only when a healthy diet in accordance with the theory of the five elements fails to reinstate health would other therapeutic measures such as acupuncture or herbs be considered. A healthy diet has always been recommended over the course of the history of German medicine. There have been various approaches, ranging from Hildegard von Bingen to wholemeal diets to F. X. Mayr regimens. Some swear by raw food diets or the M. O. Bruker wholefoods diet, others vouch for lactovegetarian diets, five element diets, alkaline diets, metabolic typing, or metabolic balancing. And this list is not exhaustive by any means. There are many truths and many roads that lead to health. It is worth experimenting to find out what kind of diet helps you to feel good and to get well.

Enjoy your food and enjoy good health. Here is a simple, short summary of what we have covered.

Summary

> Eat plenty of fruit, vegetables and whole grain produce. Choose vegetable oils. Avoid refined sugar and white flour (if you have a sweet tooth use fructose or stevia as a sweetener). Most importantly, eat foods in their most natural state. Margarine, for example, is less natural than butter, UHT milk is less natural than fresh milk, canned food may be well preserved but is not as full of life as fresh produce.

Incidentally, every study carried out has shown that animals, when offered a choice between organic and conventionally grown food, choose organic food. You will find that and other revealing facts in Hans-Ulrich Grimm's book *Die Ernährungsfalle* [The Nutritional Trap, only available in German]. This informative reference book reveals how the food industry manipulates our food and reveals the various additives used to preserve, flavour or add colour to the food that stands on the shelves of our supermarkets. Among these additives are wood shavings, fish offal, moulds and artificial 'designer' substances. A number of these additives are known to have pathogenic effects and many products contain a combination of such substances. I quote (in translation) the first part of the section on 'Modified Starches' to give you an example of the possible effects on your health (pp. 321–2):

> Modified starch is one of the newly-created designer substances not found in nature. It was 'tailor made' by suppliers for the needs of the food industry. Modified starch can be found in a number of health and diet products, in industrial muesli for example, and in a number of foods for children. It causes spikes in blood-sugar levels and the sugar-regulating hormone insulin and can, as a result, disrupt the way the body processes food and regulates weight. The effect is similar to giving your child some white bread and sugar with their muesli. Modified starch can even be used in dairy products used for weaning babies (infant food).
> (Source: Hans-Ulrich Grimm, *Die Ernährungsfalle* [The Nutritional Trap] Heyne Verlag, 2010, ISBN 978-3453170742)

Modified starch is one of the ingredients found in processed foods that damages the body's endocrine system. The 'designer starch' is a fast carbohydrate with a high glycaemic index. It has an index value of 95, higher than marzipan, gummy bears and Mars bars. What that means is that modified starch quickly causes the hormone insulin, which processes sugar, to spike. That can be a contributing factor in obesity and disorders such as metabolic syndrome, and increases the risk of heart disease and diabetes. It is also thought to cause bowel cancer.

> Designer starch is an ingredient in Nestlé's Alete Jogolino Strawberry yogurt for children, Hipp's Hippness Crisp Muesli, Weight Watchers' fruit yogurts and other product ranges. Maggi's cream of mushroom soup should actually be called 'modified starch soup' because that, according to the label, is its main ingredient. You might well encounter this new ingredient in your local restaurant, canteen, or hospital. The catering firm ETO, for example, which is part of the Dr Oetker empire, adds modified starch to its egg and mushroom pancakes.
> The way food is packaged has consequences for our health. You will find important information regarding so-called softening agents by searching for the term 'plastic hormones'. I strongly suspect that food which has been lying in clear plastic packaging for a period of time has absorbed softening agents, since it has been

Information

proven that these are passed on upon contact with food. Softening agents are substances made from plastic. They disrupt the body's hormonal balance because they act in a similar way to hormones. This can cause metabolic disorders such as diabetes and obesity, as well as immune system disorders, damage to the bones and certain types of cancer. Sexual development and fertility can also be impaired.

I find that particularly worrying because plastic hormone impurities are found particularly frequently in processed baby food, dummies and children's toys. I therefore recommend: avoiding foods wrapped in plastic or in plastic film and I would urge you to prepare your own fresh baby foods. Then you know what is in it. Glass or porcelain containers can be used to store leftover food. You may not always be able to avoid giving your child a dummy. It is worth asking the retailer whether or not the dummy contains softening agents. In the long term, retailers will stock what consumers demand. Dummies and baby bottles that do not contain the disruptive hormone bisphenol A are available.

Weight problems If you have weight problems, it would be particularly useful for you to read Dr William Davis's book *Wheat Belly* (HarperCollins, 2014). It would also be worth researching other aspects of the food industry such as food additives (E numbers), children's food and artificial foods. When you have thoroughly researched everything that may be hidden in your food, it will be much easier to change to a healthy diet.

Here are a few reading suggestions to get you started:

Reading list William L. Wolcott and Trish Fahey, *The Metabolic Typing Diet* (Broadway, 2002)

Barbara Temelie, *The Five Elements Wellness Plan* (Sterling, 2003)

18.3.4. Living consciously: your energy

You have a range of different kinds of energy at your disposal. Your direct sources of energy include physical (and nervous), emotional, mental, and spiritual energy. Your time, money and possessions can also be regarded as indirect sources of energy. It is important to understand that energy always follows intention and that energy can never disappear or be destroyed, it can only be transformed. If you are clear about your goals, the flow of your energy automatically moves in this direction, taking you towards your goal. As long as you do not make a conscious decision, you will be steered by unconscious thoughts, by impressions and old belief patterns that restrict you in your thinking, often without being aware of it. You will be at the mercy of those who have set clear goals and are working to achieve them. It is comparable to being on a journey: if you are not clear about where exactly you want to go you could end up anywhere. It makes it much more likely that you will find yourself somewhere you don't want to be.

If you are unsatisfied with your life it is important to consider what your goals are. Then decide how to invest your energy to achieve them. There is little point in using violence to fight against war. Peace is a condition that can only come about and be permanently maintained if peace rules the hearts of the people involved. Angry thoughts hurled about in rage affect the universe and contribute to strife. You can only achieve peace by being peaceful within yourself. Anything else can only produce short periods of ceasefire. Anyone who has experienced this state of deep peace at least once in their lives will know that it is worth making peace with people, circumstances, or past events that have rightly aroused indignation. You can stand your ground if you prefer. But in doing so your energy is steered towards unpleasant feelings. Things become difficult if you believe that others are to blame for your bad feelings. That is not true. Your feelings are always your responsibility. *Making peace promotes healing*

Your thoughts determine how you feel and nobody else can change those thoughts. You also carry the consequences, no matter what you decide. It is important that you understand how much power you have. You really can choose your thoughts.

Thoughts are free. No one can stop your thoughts.

You lose much energy when you rant about circumstances that annoy you. When you complain, your life becomes harder. If you want things to become easier again, observe how you handle your energy. There is always plenty of energy available in the universe. So there is no reason to be trapped with a lack of energy. When you become enthusiastic about something, a great deal of energy flows into you. If a long time has passed since you felt enthusiasm and you have forgotten how it feels … *Energy drains*

... enthusiasm arises when something truly brings you joy, or when you experience a deep sense of meaning. Things may be somewhat strenuous every now and then as you work your way towards your goals but that will hardly bother you if you are being carried forward by true enthusiasm.

If you lack energy it is because you do not stand up for your own cause. Just realising this is a tremendous help if it leads to you taking responsibility for yourself again. That is the only way of becoming aware of your own power. Formulate your goals. Take well-being as an example – consider what in your life gives you a sense of well-being and what does not. Then decide to use your energy for those things that promote well-being. These can be small things woven into the fabric of your day, such as taking a ten minute break in the open air, doing a 15 minute morning exercise routine, or a jovial meet-up with friends. Do whatever increases your sense of well-being.

You may realise that your job, your home, your partner or your family do not contribute to your sense of well-being. I am not advising you to make drastic life changes here. I cannot judge your situation. But sometimes that might be necessary if you want to maintain or regain your health.

Reading suggestion   Being honest with yourself is an important first step. If you have relationship problems, I recommend you first read the books *Men Are From Mars, Women Are From Venus* by John Gray, and *Love Who You Are and It Doesn't Matter Who You Marry* by Eva-Maria Zurhorst. If you take notice of your emotions, it is possible that you will find a solution that keeps you healthy. Setting yourself the goal of increasing well-being does not mean that you may not also feel sad, angry or fearful. Such feelings can be released if you allow them to surface. If you are reluctant to perceive the emotion, the emotion you resist causes a serious loss of energy. A part of you must now constantly be engaged with the task of suppressing this unpleasant feeling. The longer these aspects of yourself are kept in this warded off state, the more energy it costs you. Dealing with such intense feelings in this way is a part of our standard defence mechanism. In other words, everyone reacts in this way. But that does not mean we should leave things as they are. It is your choice. If you want to become or remain well, one of the basic prerequisites is to accept yourself as you are – including everything you do not like about yourself and all the previously repressed emotions. Incidentally, getting to know yourself better can be very exciting. Increased energy, more happiness and better health are just a few of the results to expect. Taking a closer interest in yourself really is worth it.

How you use your time is an important issue. Do you use your time to do things that bring you joy? Or do you simply fulfil your duties, never taking the time to do what you want to do? If you feel you don't have enough time, it may help to do a quick check. There are certain things in your life you cannot do every day because you have a job or some other duty to perform. You also need to set aside a certain period aside for sleep, time for personal hygiene, and so on. Only a certain part of every 24 hours remains free to use as you please. *Time management*

The proportion of leisure time is relatively high in our industrialised society. Choose to use that in a way that is beneficial to your health by setting priorities.

Do you get enough sleep? Different people need different amounts of sleep. It is irrelevant how much sleep other people need. You should only be concerned with how much sleep you need in order to feel good, and make sure you get it. *Adequate sleep*

How much time do you need by yourself, and how much time do you want to spend with your partner and your family? How much time do you want to spend with friends, and which friends do you want to spend time with? How much time do you want to spend working on your hobby, volunteering, or on other activities? Only you can know what you really need. When you are clear on that, organise your time accordingly. Of course, it will be different if you are a single mother, an overworked freelancer, or unemployed. But everyone can organise a tailor-made time management system for themselves. If you observe the structure of your days realistically and watch out for what your heart desires, you will find opportunities to do exactly what you want, at least for a few minutes a day or a few hours a week. The joy that results from doing so can give you more energy than you can perhaps imagine at present.

The way you deal with money can also promote or endanger your health. If you are constantly spending more than you have available, you will fall into debt. That makes life difficult. The bigger the mountain of debt, the more oppressive your situation. The only solution is to get right to the bottom of things, analyse your income and your outgoings, and either increase your income by taking on additional work or look for ways to reduce your outgoings. It is also important to consider what and who you want to support with your money. Products that are ignored *Dealing with money* by consumers quickly disappear from the market. In other words, we all have the power to make sure that child labour and inhumane working practices are no longer utilised. If we only buy products that are ethically certified, the day will come when child labour no longer exists. The same is true of food produced by using cruel intensive livestock farming practices, fishing techniques that kill dolphins, wood from tropical rainforests, and so on. If, when we go shopping, we ask where a product comes from or how it was produced, we raise awareness of these issues among retailers, especially if the products end up staying on their shelves.

We can all help to make this world a better place, every day, with every pound we spend.

The way we invest our money plays an important role energetically. As long as we continue to blindly trust the banks with our money without taking any interest in what they do with it, we should not be surprised when they do as they please with it.

Do you care whether or not the funds your money is invested in contain the shares of companies that make their profits from genetic engineering, the arms trade, or outsourcing their production sites to countries which pay low wages? If you do, it is vital that you don't just look for opportunities to make a profit, but that you also decide to which companies you are happy to hand over your money. That might not always lead to huge profits, but instead, you know where you have invested your surplus energy and you can sleep with a clear conscience. Money cannot increase of its own accord – a person must produce the value that is behind it. If we can buy a cheap product or if we make a large profit in a financial transaction, someone somewhere has either been badly paid or has suffered a loss.

The question is: is it worth paying this price to increase your wealth? And don't think it is not a problem just because everyone else is doing it. Together, we all have enormous power. If we apply our energy consciously to get what we want, we can change our world very quickly indeed.

18.3.5 Living consciously: cosmetics, shoes and clothing

The skin is our biggest organ. Whatever comes into contact with it can be absorbed through the pores into the body, and especially so when we perspire. It is, therefore, important to avoid allowing harmful substances of any kind from coming into contact with the skin. Cosmetics, shoes and clothing can all be contaminated.

Harmful substances in cosmetic products

The Occupational Safety and Health Administration of the US Department of Labor found 2,083 chemicals in personal hygiene products of various kinds, 884 of which were poisonous:

146 of those can cause tumours

376 can lead to eye and skin irritation

314 can cause biological changes

218 can lead to fertility problems

(Multiples possible)

(Source: www.s-hennbach.de/gh/Infos/Schadstoffe.htm)

Reading suggestions

You can find information regarding harmful substances in cosmetic products by searching the internet. A list of harmful substances is included on www.lifestudio.info/harmful.htm – these are ingredients no one would voluntarily and knowingly want to apply to their skin. Unfortunately most conventional personal hygiene products contain such ingredients. Skin creams, shampoos, toothpastes, shaving foams, make-up, gels, liquid soaps, lotions, lip gloss, deodorants, perfumes and anything else you might have in your bathroom – they are almost certain to contain dangerous ingredients of one kind or another, usually more than just one.

The US Food and Drug Administration (FDA) has stipulated that cosmetic producers can use any ingredients and any raw materials and bring the end product onto the market without the government's approval.
(Source: www.zeitenschrift.com/magazin/40-kosmetik.ihtml: 'Although the Food and Drug Administration [FDA] classifies cosmetic articles, it does not regulate them, however hard that is to believe. As you can see from a document on the homepage of this agency [http:/vm.cfsan.fda.gov/~dms/cos-hdb1.htlm], "cosmetics producers may use any ingredients and any raw materials and bring the end product onto the market without the government's approval."')

That is truly outrageous when you consider how dangerous most of these substances are. Here are some examples taken from the article quoted above in the magazine *Zeitenschrift*:

Alpha Hydroxy Acids
These are organic acids that are formed through anaerobic respiration. Skin care products containing a-hydroxy acids attack not only the skin cells but also the skin's protective layer. This can result in long-term damage to the skin.

Aluminium (e.g. aluminium chlorohydrate)
A metallic element used in perspiration-inhibiting products (e.g. deodorants), antiseptic agents and antacids. When applied to the skin, aluminium closes the pores, thereby preventing perspiring. This stops natural detoxification through the skin. Aluminium makes its way through the skin and into the blood. Aluminium is often linked with Alzheimer's disease and breast cancer.

Collagen
An insoluble fibrous protein that cannot penetrate the skin due to its size. The collagen that is used in most skin care products is obtained from animal hides and ground chicken feet. The substance covers the skin like a film and can suffocate it.

Diethanolamine (DEA)
Also: cocamide DEA, lauramide DEA. A colourless or crystalline alcohol that is used in solvents, emulsifiers and cleansers. DEA works as a softener in skin lotions and as a moisturising agent in skin care products. When these DEAs are processed with nitrates they react with each other, possibly leading to the formation of carcinogenic nitrosamines. The most recent studies show carcinogenic potential even without nitrate bonding. DEAs also irritate the skin and mucous membranes.

Diethyl phthalate
Used as an alcohol denaturant. It is absorbed by the skin and affects its protective mechanisms. It is thought that phthalates are harmful to the liver, kidneys and the reproductive organs and they have a hormone-like effect.

Elastin with high relative molecule mass
A similar protein to collagen and a main component of elastic fibres. Elastin is acquired from animal parts. Its effect on the skin is similar to that of collagen.

Fluoride
Fluoride is an environmental pollutant that is not biodegradable. It is an industrial waste product that is officially classified as a poisonous substance by the US Environmental Protection Agency. Dr Dean Burk former head of the National Cancer Institute says: 'Fluoride causes more human cancer deaths, and causes it faster than any other chemical substance.' All toothpastes containing fluoride have been banned in Belgium.

Formaldehyde/-donors
(Such as bronidox, bronopol, diazolidinyl-urea, DMDM hydanotin, imidazolidinyl urea, 2-bromo-2-nitropropane-1,3-diol, 2,4-imidazolidinedione, 5-bromo-5-nitro-1,3-dioxane)
A colourless, poisonous gas – an irritant and carcinogenic. Formaldehyde mixed with water is used as a disinfectant, fixative, or preservative. A number of cosmetic products contain formaldehyde, especially conventional nail care products. This substance, which is thought to cause cancer, irritates mucous membranes even in small quantities and can trigger allergies. It also ages the skin.

Lanolin
A fatty substance that comes from wool, known as a skin sensitizer, that is often used in cosmetics and lotions. Skin can sometimes react allergically to lanolin, for example by breaking out in a rash. Tests carried out on lanolin in 1988 discovered that it contained 16 pesticides.

Mineral oil
Paraffin oil, for example paraffinum liquidum. Derived from crude oil (petroleum), it is used industrially as a cutting fluid and a lubricant oil. Mineral oil forms an oily film on the skin. As a result, moisture, toxins and waste substances are trapped and normal skin respiration is inhibited because oxygen cannot penetrate the skin.

Perfume (usually nitro- and polycyclic musk compounds)
Animal testing has shown some of these synthetic aroma chemicals to be carcinogenic or mutagenic. These substances accumulate in the environment and in the body and have even been detected in breast milk.

Propylene glycol
Material safety data sheets warn users to avoid contact between propylene glycol and the skin because it is a strong skin irritant (contact dermatitis) and can lead to liver abnormalities and kidney damage.

Sodium fluoride
This substance has been identified as a potential carcinogenic.

Sodium lauryl sulphate (SLS)
A harsh cleaning agent and surfactant that is used to clean garage floors, in engine lubricants, and in car-cleaning products. It is added to almost all cleaning products as a foaming agent. Sodium lauryl sulphate is considered by scientists to be a common skin allergen. It is quickly absorbed by the eyes, brain, heart and liver and is stored in those organs, potentially leading to long-term damage. Sodium lauryl sulphate can generally slow the body's healing processes and cause cataracts in adults and eye development problems in children.

Sodium laureth sulphate (SLES)
Sodium laureth sulphate is the alcoholised version (ethoxylated) form of sodium lauryl sulphate. The highly toxic compound 1,4-dioxane is formed during the ethoxylation process. 1,4-dioxane was one of the principal components of the chemical defoliant 'Agent Orange' used during the Vietnam war. 1,4-dioxane disrupts the body's hormonal balance and is suspected of being the main cause of some types of cancer. This substance is very similar to the hormone oestrogen and it is thought to increase the risk of breast cancer, endometrial (womb) cancer, stress-related illnesses, and reduced sperm production.

Sunscreens / UV filters
Substances such as 4-MBC (4-methylbenzylidene camphor), OMC (Octyl methoxycinnamate), Bp-3 (Benzophenon-3)
Bp-3 is now suspected of acting in a similar way to the female hormone oestrogen. UV filters have been detected in human breast milk and in fish. A study carried out at the University of Zurich's Institute of Pharmacology and Toxicology showed that breast cancer cells grew when five different UV filters were applied to them.

Talc
A soft, grey-green mineral substance. Inhalation can be harmful because this substance is known to be a serious carcinogenic. Talc is widely thought to be one of the main causes of ovarian cancer.

The list could go on. The question for you now is this: do you really want these things on your skin?

Fortunately we have an alternative: natural cosmetics. In addition to well-established companies such as Weleda and Dr Hauschka, there are a number of other manufacturers and seals of quality that represent various quality standards. Demeter, NaTrue, Naturland, BDIH, Ecocert, and Lacon are just some of the quality standard seals that certify the ingredients used. There is also the Leaping Bunny seal and the IHTK seal that stand for 'animal-free testing'. If you want to be sure that you are really buying natural cosmetics, read the packaging very carefully. Some companies want to take advantage of the organic trend by advertising their products as being 'organic' or 'natural' despite the fact that they actually contain many chemicals. You will find detailed information regarding the individual quality seals for natural cosmetic products on: www.ecco-verde.co.uk/categories/certificates-labels.

The alternative: natural cosmetics

Shoes and clothing

Clothes should look good and cost as little as possible. Production costs must be kept low. For this reason, most of our clothes are produced in Southeast Asia. European retailers hardly ever check how wool, leather and other raw materials are treated there. As a result, a range of substances that are not approved for use in clothes and shoes in Europe end up, via cheap imports, on your skin. More than 7,000 chemicals are used in clothes production processes. Here are just a few.

Azo dyes can release carcinogenic substances once they have been absorbed by the body. That is why the use of azo dyes in clothes was banned in Germany in 1966. They have not been banned in Asia, where they continue to be used because they are cheap and are good dyes.

Chrome compounds, which are often found in leather products, are known to be carcinogenic.

In Germany, **dispersion dyes** that are needed to dye synthetic fibres may be present in clothes up to certain limits even though they tend to cause contact allergies.

Potassium dichromate is used to tan leather. Residues, in cheap shoes for example, can cause allergies in the skin of the feet. Worryingly, animal testing has shown that the substance has mutagenic and carcinogenic effects.

Pentachlorophenol (PCP) kills mildew. Although its production and use have been banned in Germany since the 1980s, PCP continues to be present in imported textiles. PCP can lead to chlorine acne and nerve damage, and in high doses can lead to high blood pressure and heart failure.

Formaldehyde is used to prevent fabrics from crumpling. Animal testing showed that it has mutagenic and carcinogenic effects. Clothes advertised as 'no-iron' or 'wrinkle-free' almost certainly contain formaldehyde.
(Source: www.konsumo.de/news/104880-Azofarbstoffe%20Kleidung%20Allergien%20Haut%20Reizung)

Organotin compounds are extremely poisonous. Tributyltin (TBT) is used more widely in clothes than mono- and dibutyltin. (Source: www.medizininfo.de/hautundhaar/kleidung/gift.htm) TBT is absorbed by the skin and deposited in the liver and kidneys, which can lead to serious liver and kidney disorders, and weakens the immune system. In addition, TBT interferes with hormones. This increases the risk of sterility in men and can cause women to take on male characteristics. TBT was found in Nike's Borussia Dortmund football shirts. Children who support Borussia Dortmund and who want to wear their team's shirt are at particular risk because they perspire when playing and running around, and the skin's pores open wide. Many other teams in the UK, and throughout Europe and the rest of the world, play in Nike football shirts.

TBT is still used in Germany to hinder the fouling on ships' hulls. It has been proven that about 140 snail species in the North Sea are now in danger of extinction as a result.

Good advice is expensive, according to an old German saying. But it is worth it because it is good. The same is true when buying products: quality comes at a price. A piece of clothing that only costs a few pounds cannot have been made using quality materials and the workers cannot have been paid a fair wage. It can also be assumed that cheap clothing contains harmful substances. The 'Arte' TV documentary 'Gift – unser tägliches Risiko' [Poison – our daily hazard] by Inge Altmeier and Reinhard Hornung (broadcast 27/07/2010) revealed that 99% of our clothes are contaminated with poisons. The programme featured people who have become ill because of their clothes and shoes. In addition, the programme showed a worker in Bangladesh wading barefoot, up to his ankles in azo dyes. It is shocking to learn that a label with the declaration 'organic cotton' is sewn onto the t-shirts at the request of the European contractor. More 'organic cotton' is sold worldwide than is grown in the first place. This is why quality standard seals are so important. The Öko-Tex-100 seal is well established. It only allows the use of harmful substances up to a certain limit and therefore offers a certain minimum standard. The environmental impact of production is not taken into consideration when awarding the seal. The GOTS seal has stricter constraints: it is only awarded when at least 90% natural fibres from environmentally friendly production processes are used. Other quality seals for organically-produced and socially-responsible clothing include Demeter, Naturland and IVN. Producers such as Engel, Maus and hessnatur have been certified by GOTS. Due to increased demand, large retail chains such as C&A and Wal-Mart now also offer some ranges that comply with the new international GOTS standard.

If you need to buy new clothes, look for these certification seals. Whatever you decide, I would advise you to wash every piece of new clothing before wearing it for the first time. If it does not come with a seal that you trust, you might want to leave it to soak overnight. If the water becomes dyed it is worth soaking again until the article no longer loses colour. I would then recommend you wash it a number of times in your washing machine. In my opinion, articles of clothing will largely be free of harmful substances when they have been washed seven times. I wear my clothes for as long as possible before buying new ones because there is only a very small chance that clothes that have been worn and washed often still contain harmful substances. That is good for me and good for the environment.

The effect of most poisons creeps stealthily upon us, accumulating slowly over the years. In such matters, prevention really is better than a cure. I, in any case, only want water, soap and organically produced textiles on my skin, and when necessary good oils or natural cosmetics.

18.3.6 Living consciously: your home and workplace

Depending on the intensity and duration of exposure, geopathic stress and electrosmog can have a harmful effect on the human body. In the past, people had a sense for energetically powerful sites and they carried out their religious rituals there. Churches were usually built in such places. Old farmhouses often stand in such propitious places. As the density of the population increases, less and less consideration is given to such matters. Today, many earth dislocation lines, generally known as water veins in the past, run directly through people's bedrooms or even their beds. Long-term exposure to geopathic stress can lead to illnesses and can hinder the healing process. If you do not experience an improvement in your health despite your best efforts, it might be worth asking an experienced dowser to work on your home. Sometimes it is just a bed that needs to be moved. Sometimes lines and networks cross and overlap, leading to geopathic stress in specific areas of homes and bedrooms. I have developed the 'Sei gut behütet zu Hause' [Well protected at home] glass orb especially to neutralise harmful radiation within a defined area of effectiveness. It can transform geopathic stresses of all kinds, as well as electrosmog produced by transmitters and electronic equipment such as computers, TVs, cordless (DECT) telephones, mobile phones, and so on. There is also a version for the workplace, where electrosmog pollution is often even higher. I have designed a smaller glass orb especially for travel: it is designed to help you deal with all the changes and adjustments that leisure and business travel entails. What is more, it neutralises the harmful geopathic stress and electrosmog as does the larger 'Well protected at home' orb. If you are interested, you will find all the relevant information on the website

Neutralising radiation

www.informierteGlobuli.de

Further reading

Ulrike Banis, *Geopathic Stress – and what you can do about it* (Comed, 2003)

Jane Thurnell-Read, *Geopathic Stress: How Earth Energies Affect our Lives* (Element, 1995)

Holistically oriented doctors regard the impact of high-frequency microwave radiation as being even more worrying than geopathic stress. Long-term international studies have proved that mobile phone radiation causes harm when people are exposed over periods of years. As a result, the Ärztekammer Wien [Association of Viennese Doctors] has issued this advice for mobile phone use:

Ten rules for mobile phone use

- Use your mobile phone as little as possible and when you do use it keep calls short. Use landlines or VoIP. Children and teenagers under 16 should only carry mobiles for use in emergencies.
- Keep the phone away from the body (at arm's length) while the call is connecting.
- Do not make calls in the car, train or bus – the radiation is stronger.
- Hold the phone as far away from the body as possible when sending text messages.
- Buy a mobile phone that has an external antenna and a low SAR-value.
- Do not keep your mobile in your trouser pocket – the radiation could affect men's fertility.
- At home, switch off your mobile and use the landline.
- Do not play games on your mobile.
- When using headsets or integrated hands-free equipment, keep the mobile as far away from the body as possible (e.g. in your outer skirt pocket or handbag).
- WLAN and UMTS, in particular, lead to high long-term exposure.

Find more information on the dangers of mobile phone radiation, as well as a comprehensive list of studies and further reading, in the following article:
http://www.lef.org/magazine/mag2007/aug2007_report_cellphone_radiation_01.htm

The German website www.kinder-und-handys.de/erkenntnisse reports the results of various scientific studies that prove the harmful effect of mobile phone radiation on human health. The main health problems caused are brain damage resulting from the opening of the blood-brain

Crystal orbs

barrier, exhaustion, headaches in children, damage to sperm and embryos, and increased risk of cancer demonstrated in DNA bond disruption. Cordless phones with DECT technology constantly transmit high-frequency waves from the base station and they can have a harmful effect on your health. It is therefore worth getting rid of old cordless DECT phones and buying a new-generation cordless phone. Fortunately, analogue phones are almost universally the standard again. I have programmed crystal orbs to transform all the harmful frequencies transmitted by modern technological devices so that the radiation is made harmless within an effective area of 8 to 30 metres (depending on the size of the orb). These are the same orbs as those designed to neutralise geopathic stress. You will find more information on: www.informierteGlobuli.de.

Energy-saving bulbs

So-called energy-saving bulbs come with a host of disadvantages – problems that manufacturers, retailers, and the media rarely mention. Energy-saving lamps emit pulsing, high-frequency radiation fields that are known to be particularly harmful biologically.

> 'Only a small percentage of light serves to help us see with the eyes. A much larger percentage is responsible for the regulation of important metabolic processes and life rhythm, for the production and regulation of hormones and vitamins, and has an important effect on the immune system and the mind, on the blood and hair.'
> Source: *Apotheken-Umschau* (June 2008)

The building biologist Wolfgang Maes, in an article entitled 'Hinters Licht geführt: Energiesparlampen' [Energy-saving Lamps: Pulling the Wool over our Eyes], writes:

Electrosmog

'... energy-saving bulbs produce far more electrosmog than is allowed for PC monitors, they emit harmful substances, production is energy-intensive, they contain poisonous materials that should be disposed of as toxic waste, but are usually disposed of with the rest of the household rubbish – a few hundred kilograms of mercury goes to poison the environment in Germany alone each year.'

This list is not exhaustive by any means. The Heidelberg doctor Alexander Wunsch explains in his lecture 'Ja! zur Glühlampe – ein Plädoyer für ein gesundes Leuchtmittel' [Yes to the incandescent bulb! A plea for healthy lamps] (2007):

'No lamp produces a light spectrum that is so similar to the sun as the incandescent bulb ... the sun and the incandescent bulb produce a continuous spectrum ... Light from fluorescent lamps, that is from energy-saving bulbs, causes reactions in the body that can lead to the onset of a number of the diseases of civilisation ... To recommend the use of energy-saving lamps on the basis of reduced energy bills, without taking the hidden costs of production and disposal into consideration, leads to a completely distorted picture.'

Wolfgang Maes, in his speech at the 1st International Lighting Design Congress (10/07) in London, described the ban on incandescent bulbs as a state-decreed assault on its citizens as long as no comparable bulbs are available. 'Energy-saving lamps are not the solution. Many people know this from their own experience. When placed close to the head, they cause headaches and a feeling of pressure, light-headedness, vibration, and lead to concentration problems and eye problems.'
(Source: www.buergerwelle-schweiz.org, June 2007).

I personally find the light produced by energy-saving lamps unpleasant. I disposed of them after trying them out for the first time because I did not feel comfortable using them. Perhaps there is a better light than the incandescent bulb but the energy-saving bulb is not it.

Building in a biological way would be very advantageous because the spaces we live in surround us like a third skin.
We inhale and absorb, at least in part, whatever is emitted and released into our surroundings. The danger posed by certain substances only becomes apparent many years later, as was the case with asbestos. If the producers of building materials and windows are to make an effort to be more environmentally friendly, we as customers have to put pressure on them to do so. The choice of goods available will only improve if we demand good quality and not just low prices.

18.3.7 Living consciously: vaccinations

Many people know that vaccinations can lead to complications, leaving children with vaccine injury in some circumstances. However, only a few people know that there is no proof that any vaccination really protects against the disease it is meant to make us immune to.

Vaccinations only produce increased antibody counts. That is enough for a substance to be approved as a vaccine.

There is no requirement that clinical studies should provide proof that vaccinations immunise against a disease. Such proof does not exist.

The World Health Organisation carried out a large field study in Southern India between 1968 and 1971. About 400,000 people in the province of Madras were given the BCG vaccine, another 400,000 were not given the vaccine. Two test areas in the province of Madras had been chosen in advance to form two groups of roughly equal size. Then the whole population of one area, apart from infants below the age of one year, was vaccinated while the population in the other area was not. In 1979 the WHO published the first interim report: eleven years after the study started, there had been considerably more cases of TB among the vaccinated population than there had been in the unvaccinated area. The unvaccinated people had a lower chance of becoming ill with TB.

In other words, the TB vaccination increased people's risk of becoming ill with TB.
(Source: Dr Gerhard Buchwald, *Der Rückgang der Schwindsucht trotz 'Schutzimpfung'* [The Decline of TB despite 'preventative' Vaccination] (Hirthammer Verlag, 2002).

Shocking statistics regarding outbreaks of foot and mouth disease in Europe in 1966 and 1988 show that European countries that have forced vaccination programmes suffered significantly higher numbers of outbreaks; countries that did not carry out annual blanket vaccination programmes had significantly fewer cases of foot and mouth. In verifiable cases, it became clear that foot and mouth disease was introduced from countries that vaccinated against the disease. Countries that did not have forced vaccination programmes were free of the disease for many years.
(Source: K. Strohmaier, *Wie kann Europa frei von Maul- und Klauenseuche werden und bleiben?* [How can Europe be rid of foot and mouth disease forever?], lecture at the Vakzineinstitut Basel, March 1989)

Tetanus vaccinations do not offer any guarantee against falling ill with that disease – on the contrary: Simone Delarue, the author of the book *Impfschutz – Irrtum oder Lüge* [Vaccinations – Mistake or Deceit?], shows how tetanus vaccinations in the French army failed to reduce the numbers succumbing to the disease. In 1,000 cases, the number was just as high during the Second World War as it was during the First

World War when no vaccinations were given. In contrast, the Greek army, which did not vaccinate its soldiers, had one-seventh the number of cases of tetanus. The decline of tetanus in Europe (isolated cases appear, in some years there is not a single case in Germany) can be attributed to improved standards of hygiene.

Tetanus, like other infectious diseases, is more common is Asian and African countries where unfavourable living conditions such as poverty, famine and contaminated water supplies, are present. Tetanus vaccinations have no effect in western countries: this is seen in a graph depicting the development of tetanus in Germany between 1962 and 1990.
(Source: Federal Statistical Office in Wiesbaden. The widespread tetanus vaccination programme slows down the elimination of tetanus.)

About 15 deaths are reported in connection with tetanus vaccinations each year.
(Source: *impf-report*, Tolzin Verlag, Edition 48/49, Nov/Dec 2008)

Measles vaccinations offer just as little protection. It is common for those vaccinated against measles to fall ill with the disease. In 1986 there was an epidemic in schools in a district of Wisconsin despite a vaccination rate of 94%. Among 218 patients who were confirmed to have the disease, 182 (83.4%) had been vaccinated in accordance with the standard procedure, 13 (6%) had never been vaccinated and 21 (10%) had only been given one vaccination in their first year.

In the Canadian provinces of British Columbia, Manitoba and Nova Scotia in 1986, out of 5,575 measles patients, 60% had been vaccinated, 28% had not been vaccinated, and the vaccination history of the remaining 12% was not known.
(Source: Simone Delarue, *Impfschutz – Irrtum oder Lüge*)

It appears that vaccination increases the risk of becoming ill with exactly the disease the vaccination is meant to protect you from. To speak of immunisation is misleading. I would never have myself vaccinated because I regard it as grievous bodily harm of the highest order.

It is not simply that it increases your risk of catching the disease in question. Vaccination also increases your chances of suffering from other side effects – as the statistics clearly demonstrate.

One vaccination programme had particularly devastating consequences for children in Guinea-Bissau. Aaby et al. discovered in one long-term study that **children vaccinated against diphtheria, tetanus and whooping cough had a mortality rate twice as high as that of unvaccinated children**. For five years, the study observed 15,000 mothers whose children had been born between 1990 and 1996. At 4.7%, the child mortality rate was very high in Guinea-Bissau, probably as a result of poor living conditions. But after the administration of the triple vaccination, child mortality rose to 10.5% among those vaccinated – more than double. (Source: Kristensen, Aaby and Jensen, 'Routine vaccinations and child survival: follow-up study in Guinea-Bissau, West Africa', *British Medical Journal* 2000; 321: 1435–1441).

An English cohort study (McKeever et al., 'Vaccination and Allergic Disease: A Birth Cohort Study', June 2004, Vol. 94, No. 6, *American Journal of Public Health*) examined the data of about 30,000 children born between 1988 and 1999 for a possible connection between vaccinations and allergies. The risk of asthma was up to 14 times lower for unvaccinated children and the risk of eczema was up to 9 times lower. A New Zealand study came to a similar conclusion in 1992: the risk of asthma there was 5 times lower for unvaccinated children, the risk of skin outbreaks 2.5 times lower, and the risk of hyperactivity 8 times lower. A study in Salzburg surveyed 374 families with a total of 572 children and discovered no asthma among unvaccinated children; only 4% had atopic eczema (10–20% in general population), and only 3% had allergies (25% in general population).
A Swedish study came to the conclusion that vaccinations, antibiotics and antipyretic medicines increase the risk of allergies in children. (Source: *impf-report*, 3/2005, www.impf-report.de, 'Geimpfte – Ungeimpfte: Wer ist gesünder?' [Vaccinated – Unvaccinated: Who is healthier?])

There are many reasons not to be vaccinated against Swine flu. First of all, there is no proof of efficacy in the sense that those vaccinated enjoy better health. There is no proof for any of the approved pandemic vaccinations. It seems unlikely that this situation will change – regarding the new influenzas or any other vaccinations.

In a January 2011 report, the Finnish government openly admitted that *State* the Swine flu vaccine can cause severe nerve damage, such as narco- *admissions* lepsy, hallucinations and mental breakdowns. The Finnish government *of harmful* announced that it was prepared to offer free lifelong healthcare to the *effects* 79 children who became incurably ill as a result of the Swine flu vaccine. Despite this, there are no calls for a worldwide withdrawal of the vaccine. The vaccination lobby is skilfully but misleadingly interpreting statistics from selected studies in an attempt to cover up the fact that flu vaccines not only cause serious side effects but that they are also completely useless.

Here is one example:

In October 2011, *The Lancet*, one of the most renowned medical research journals, published a study on the efficacy and effectiveness of flu vaccines, which allegedly comes to the conclusion that the flu vaccine is up to 60% effective. (Source: M. T. Osterholm et al., 'Efficacy and effectiveness of influenza vaccines: a systematic review and meta-analysis', *The Lancet: Infectious Diseases*, published online 26 October 2011).

Such claims are only possible when you fiddle with the numbers. These are the real statistics: of 13,095 unvaccinated people, only 2.7% contracted the flu virus. That leaves 97.3% who did not become ill. In comparison, the vaccination could only prevent the disease in 1.5% of the vaccinated people. Even these statistics appear questionable to me since all clinical studies of large population groups until now have shown that vaccination increases the risk of contracting the disease vaccinated against.

Read a thorough and illuminating analysis of *The Lancet* study mentioned above, and the statistical tricks used in it, in Mike Adams' article 'Shock vaccine study reveals influenza vaccines only prevent the flu in 1.5 out of 100 adults (not 60% as you've been told)', available here: http://www.naturalnews.com/033998_influenza_vaccines_effectiveness.html (27/10/11).

Even the European Parliament criticises the waste of public funds linked to the new influenzas.

Deutsches Ärzteblatt (Vol. 107, Issue 23, 11/06/2010) reports that the European Parliament's Health Committee published a report on 04/06/2010 complaining that the WHO and European healthcare institutions refused to publish the names and conflicts of interest of those who were involved in making the recommendations on how to deal with the pandemic. The document passed by the European Parliament criticises a lack of transparency in the decision-making process and expresses misgivings regarding the influence the pharmaceutical industry has on those decisions. The way the WHO and EU institutions and governments dealt with the new influenza (A/H1N1-pandemic) led to a waste of public money and stoked unreasonable fears with regard to the health risks.

I cannot go into detail regarding each and every vaccination here – that is beyond the scope of this book. If you want to learn more or seek further advice, start with this list of recommended books and websites.

Dr Gerhard Buchwald, *Vaccination: A Business Based on Fear* (Books on Demand, 1994) ISBN 978-3833401626

Kate Birch, *Vaccine Free: Prevention and Treatment of Infectious Contagious Disease with Homeopathy* (CreateSpace) ISBN 978-1482789607

Harris L. Coulter and Barbara L. Fisher, *A Shot in the Dark* (Avery, 1991) ISBN 978-0895294630

Harris L. Coulter, *Vaccination, Social Violence and Criminality: The Medical Assault on the American Brain* (North Atlantic Books, 1990) ISBN 978-1556430848

Viera Scheibner, *Vaccination: 100 Years of Orthodox Research Shows that Vaccines Represent a Medical Assault on the Immune System* (V. Scheibner) ISBN 978-0646151243

Websites:
www.vaccineinjury.info
www.jabs.org.uk

To this day, no vaccine has been proven, as far as I am aware, to immunise the patient from the disease for which it is administered. The few studies that are available show the opposite. Moreover, vaccination increases the risk of allergies and even the risk of child mortality.

What good is all this? Anyone who has read this and still wants to be vaccinated is doing so on their own responsibility.

But what can you do if you do not want to vaccinate yourself or your child?

There is no compulsory vaccination in Germany or the UK. Nurseries, schools and other institutions have no right to demand that you or your child be vaccinated. You can find numerous arguments to justify your position in the reading material above and through support groups on the internet.

If you live in a country where compulsory vaccinations are enforced I would urge you to start campaigning for a change in the law.

Your health in your hands

There is much you can do to improve your health. The most important thing is to understand that you are 100% responsible for yourself – and not just in terms of your health. Everything you think and do (or neglect to do) has consequences for you and the people around you. And there are consequences for everything you set in motion or fail to set in motion. Only you can decide what is good for you because other people have different standards and habits, depending on their upbringing, their beliefs and their life experiences. Every person is an unique individual. If a doctor tells you that a certain medication has been well tolerated by everyone who has taken it so far, that is of little help to you if you happen to be the unlucky one in 10,000 who is unable to tolerate it. It takes some courage to stand by your beliefs regarding what you feel is good for you and what is not. This may not always make you popular but if you want to be healthy, standing up for yourself is an absolute must. If you try to please everybody, you are fighting a losing battle.

If you are no longer used to listening to your inner voice and don't even know what you actually want, it is always good to listen to your first impulse. For example, a colleague asks you whether you have time tonight to complete some urgent work for him and your first thought is 'No!' because you have something important planned for that evening. Then your head intervenes, raising doubts such as 'I can't say no to him', 'He's often helped me in the past', 'He'll think me ungrateful' or the like. So you say yes. In that situation, you neither act honestly towards yourself or your colleague. Doing something you don't want to do will not help to improve your mood or to increase your sense of well-being. Try to listen to your inner voice – it can usually be heard clearly in the first impulse. If you want to get in touch with your inner voice on a deeper level, I recommend the following meditation. Practice this by yourself if you are in good mental health and do not take any psychoactive medications or drugs. If you are unsure, it is better to practice under the supervision of an experienced meditation teacher. If you decide to try the meditation, I wish you all the best with it.

> Sit or lie back in a comfortable position.
> Close your eyes.
> Breathe in and out deeply three times.
> When exhaling, imagine that all your burdens and worries flow out of you. Mentally install a shower of light above your head. This shower of light pours a gentle purifying and healing light over you. Now visualise a room in your heart in the centre of your chest. Your reach it via a staircase. You furnish the room so that you feel at home there. Enjoy your time there. Your heart-room offers limitless possibilities. Sit by the seaside, in a meadow, in the mountains, watch a sunset, or look at a beautifully furnished house. Create what you want to see. Experiment and change things around. If it feels good, it is good. When you feel completely relaxed, ask your question, for example 'Is it wise for me to do X?' Wait, and listen to the answer your heart gives you. The first thing you hear is true. Your head will not have censored the first impulse you feel. Even just a few seconds later, the censor will probably cut in, and the fears it gives rise to will possibly drag you down to a state of despair.
> If you have never meditated before, it is better at first to practice with questions that do not involve important life decisions. You will have time to become familiar with the method so that you will be more adept at it when you need to use it under stress.

Meditation

Once you have discovered what it is you really want, the second step follows. Say it or do it. In doing so, you take responsibility for yourself and your health. I cannot promise you that this will always be easy. But I can reassure you that, over time and with practice, it will become easier and you will experience things you have never experienced before. Then see how you feel and, if necessary, adjust your course.

If you would like to try other meditations, there is a range of exercises available on CDs; these exercises can be done at home. Why not take a look, and tackle some?

Aside from meditation, there are other methods that can assist you to establish deeper contact with your body and your feelings through awareness-refining techniques; these include autogenic training, Alexander technique, Feldenkrais, yoga, qi gong, shiatsu, zilgrei, voice and breath work.

This book contains a wealth of ideas and information that should put you in a position to make decisions that serve your health. I have written this book according to the best of my knowledge and conscience. It contains the fruit of Jim Humble's work with MMS over many years, the results of my own use of MMS, and the results of other self-responsible users whom I have supervised, as well as empirical insights gained from my medical practice. Insofar, this book is a reflection of my view of truth, as my level of knowledge stands today. Since I am constantly developing and learning, in a few years time my truth may be a different one. I cannot guarantee that I would write the same book in three years' time. But I can assure you that everything I have written here represents the fruit of decades of practical medical experience. Only you can decide whether it resonates with you. Doctors can provide valuable support but healing takes place within or not at all. If a person has to swallow a range of tablets every day, possibly for the rest of his life, to alleviate or eliminate his symptoms, that suggests to me that that person is still far from healthy. The symptoms of disease have simply been suppressed by medication and are therefore currently not troubling the patient. But in the long term it will be even harder to bring the body back to a state of health because the body's attempt to provide an outlet for a deeper problem has been inhibited. Would you say that an aeroplane is in a good state of repair if a flashing warning light has been taped over? That would make me uncomfortable and I would not think the aeroplane fit to fly. Diseases are the body's warning lights. They indicate that something is not quite right. If you want to find out what is missing, it is vital that you become actively involved. You must at least have the intention of becoming well, of supporting the physical body in the best possible way, and of letting go of emotional burdens, so that you can return to a state in which the body, emotions, mind and spirit are in harmony again. Sometimes all you need to do is to change a couple of habits that are causing you problems.

Whatever you need to do to get well can only work if you are prepared to do it. And my truth does not necessarily need to be yours. You can, of course, take whatever information you find useful and implement it in your life while rejecting the remainder. That was always the intention of this book. I want to show you possibilities and choices. You decide what to do with that information. Do what you consider to be suitable. Listen to your internal voice until you become clear regarding what the correct decision is for you.

You are responsible for your health, whether you accept that responsibility or not. It is better that you consciously assume responsibility. Otherwise it is as if you are driving in traffic without acknowledging the rules of the road, as if you were simply refusing to take notice of them.

Unfortunately, that does not protect you from problems. Just as a free-flowing traffic system requires us to observe some basic rules, so too does a life of health and well-being.

The most important of these rules is that you take care of yourself, respect yourself, and set priorities in accordance with this.

If you then boldly set about cleaning up your life – and that is sometimes necessary both internally and externally – you re-establish the order that allows your physical body to remain or become healthy. That can be the beginning of a happy and fulfilled life – a life of harmony within you, and between you and others. Everyone carries the seeds of healing within themselves. If the information I have presented here helps you to reach that place, I will be very happy. And on that note, I wish you all the best and very good health.

Dr Antje Oswald

ABOUT THE AUTHOR

Dr Antje Oswald, born 1960 in Hamburg, specialist in general practice, homeopathy and psychotherapy, worked at the August-Weihe-Institute of Homeopathic Medicine in Detmold. Since 1990, she has worked in her own private practice as a classical homeopathic doctor in Detmold.

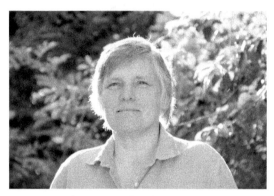

From 1986 to 2002, Dr Oswald regularly trained homeopathic doctors at the 'Detmolder Wochen' seminars and at other training institutions.

Over the last twelve years, she has been predominantly using kinesiology as a diagnostic and therapeutic tool and has been offering kinesiology courses since 2003: www.kinesiologie-kolleg.de.

In 2008, she, along with Christiane Brendel and Kerstin Depping, established a company that produces and sells energetically imprinted globules and crystal orbs: www.informierteGlobuli.de.

She was involved with the 'German Society for the Promotion of Natural Healing' for over 25 years as a member of the editorial board of *Homöopathie-aktuell,* where she also occasionally published articles. She was also heavily involved with the production of the documentary film *Homöopathie: Wer? Wo? Wie? Was?* [Homeopathy: Who? Where? How? What?] which offered an overview of the situation of homeopathy and natural healing in Germany and Europe.

To achieve her aim of understanding the complex human essence in the most holistic way possible, Dr Oswald has felt it necessary to continue to train in a variety of western and eastern healing methods. Her main concern is to encourage her patients to rediscover the potential that lies within them and to mobilise their own healing resources so that they can recover their health in a natural way.

In *The MMS Handbook*, she draws on her many years of experience to offer you a wealth of practical tips. It is her first book.

APPENDIX

Appendix

Directory of health practitioners and advisors with experience of MMS

This appendix lists doctors, alternative health practitioners, dentists, veterinarians, healers and health advisors who have experience of MMS use and who are prepared to supervise patients as they take MMS on their own responsibility.

You can contact these practitioners to arrange an appointment with them. Such consultations are, of course, subject to a charge and these costs must be met by the patient. On no account is it possible for these colleagues to give medical advice by email or phone if they have never met you personally. That is forbidden by law in many countries. Neither is it possible for them to prescribe MMS since it is only approved for use as a water disinfectant.

Those included on this list are practicing their profession within the legal parameters of their respective countries. That means you can make an appointment to see them, ask them any questions you may have regarding MMS, and learn about the opportunities and risks it may entail. They can show you how MMS is used and you can even take MMS at that doctor or practitioner's clinic, or be treated with it in some other way, for example to disinfect parts of the skin or mucous membrane. All this is possible if you decide to take MMS on your own responsibility after having been made aware that MMS is not an officially approved medication.

This list includes all those who wrote to us stating their occupational title and affirming that they were happy to be included. Many thanks to everyone who agreed to this.

Jim Humble has recently started to offer personal consultations (in English).

The price of a consultation currently (January 2015) stands at US$ 200 and can be conducted by appointment via Skype, email or by phone. See www.jimhumble.biz for more details.

Since the publisher was not aware of any other UK or US doctors or alternative practitioners who work with MMS at the time the English version of *The MMS Handbook* went to press, for now this list only contains contact details for practitioners and doctors in Germany, Austria and Switzerland. If you are a doctor or alternative practitioner with experience of working with MMS and you would like to publish your details in this book, please contact us at: info@daniel-peter-verlag.de

Postcode Area 1

Martina Willing
Bioenergetics Practitioner
Am Neuendorfer Sand 2 b
14770 Brandenburg
Phone: 0049 (0) 3381/301033
Mobile: 0049 (0) 1577 920 11 72
m.willing-vitalineum@t-online.de

Ursula Williger
Alternative Health Practitioner
Kyritzer Str. 1
16909 Wittstock
Phone: 0049 (0) 3394/43 31 36

Max Zimmermann
Alternative Health Practitioner
Lange Straße 22
17192 Waren
Phone: 0049 (0) 3991/179 73 33,
Mobile: 0049 (0) 151 22 88 72 43
www.max-zimmermann-heilpraxis.de
info@max-zimmermann-heilpraxis.de

Renate Lübbert
Alternative Health Practitioner
Moorbrinker Weg 41
19057 Schwerin
Phone: 0049 (0) 385/207 12 26
renate.luebbert@gmx.de

Postcode Area 2

Bettina Weck
Healer
21255 Tostedt
Phone: 0049 (0) 4182/28 71 68
www.orasi-alluba.de
bettina.weck@goldmail.de

Energy Healer
Anika Trebert
Niederkögt-Nord 7
21756 Osten
Phone: 0049 (0) 163 751 05 28

Rudi Senfleben
Alternative Health Practitioner
Lübecker Str. 124
22087 Hamburg
Phone: 0049 (0) 40/251 34 00
Fax: 040/254 39 13
info@senfleben.de

Barbara Berends
Health Advisor
Mergelstr. 14
26725 Emden
Phone: 0049 (0) 4921/23347
barbara.berends@web.de

Tierärztliches Institut für
angewandte Kleintiermedizin
Rahlstedter Straße 156
22143 Hamburg
Phone: 0049 (0) 40/677 21 44
www.tieraerzte-hamburg.com
HamburgVets@aol.com

Postcode Area 3

Joachim Andree
Alternative Health Practitioner
Marktstr. 34
30880 Laatzen
Phone: 0049 (0) 511/82 73 12
joachim-andree@t-online.de

Anja Bewig
In der Renne 7
31032 Betheln
Phone: 0049 (0) 151 704 18 267
www.vitalscreen-hanover.de
info@homoepatie-akupunktur-tiere.de

Dr. med. Ingo Rudolf
Specialist in Neurology,
Homeopathy
Hoffmannstr. 6a
32105 Bad Salzuflen
Phone: 0049 (0) 5222/807 56 90
info@ingo-rudolf.de

Tierheilpraxis MAYA
Veterinarian Practice
32699 Extertal
Phone: 0049 (0) 5262/99 55 95

Appendix

GP Specialising in Homeopathy and
Psychotherapy
Dr. med. Luise Stolz
Schorlemerstr. 32
33098 Paderborn
Phone: 0049 (0) 5251/879 33 33

Institut für Strukturelle Integration
Physiotherapist
Iris Huerkamp-Brown
Kanzler-Wippermann-Str. 13
33100 Paderborn
Phone: 0049 (0) 5251/879 11 22
www.structurings.com

Physiotherapy and Natural Healing
Clinic
Wioletta Janiak
Conrad-von-Soest Str. 2 a
34537 Bad Wildungen
Phone: 0049 (0) 5621/3038
www.ganzheitlichemedizin-janiak.de
wra.janiak@online.de

Jörg Loskant Heim
Health Advisor and
Physiotherapist
Frankfurter Straße 146
36043 Fulda
Phone: 0049 (0) 661/380 00 240
love@kamasha.de

Praxis „Osteopathie berührt"
Physiotherapy and
Osteopathy
Melanie Slabon
Im langen Feld 3
36154 Hosenfeld
Phone: 0049 (0) 6650/91 84 40

Rainer Taufertshöfer
Alternative Health Practitioner
Prema Seva Naturheilpraxis
Waldwinkel 22
37603 Holzminden-Neuhaus
Phone: 0049 (0) 5536/235 30 90
Mobil 01520 170 10 75
www.prema-seva-naturheilpraxis.de
heilpraktiker@prema-seva-naturheilpraxis.de

German School for Alternative
Health Practitioners Braunschweig
Susanne Thieme
Nordstrasse 13
38106 Braunschweig
Phone: 0049 (0) 531/480 39 499
www.tcm-bs.de
info@tcm-bs.de

Heikje Roscher-Schramm
Heilpraxis PASO Heilpraktikerin
Hauptstr. 54
38518 Gifhorn
Phone: 0049 (0) 5371 93 83 93
heros.c@gmx.de

Postcode Area 4

Claudia Gillmann
Alternative Health Practitioner
Rommelsmaar 15
41238 Mönchengladbach
Phone: 0049 (0) 2166/83694
Sphinx_cg@web.de

Bea Schönfeldt
Alternative Health Practitioner
Berglehne 33
42281 Wuppertal
Phone: 0049 (0) 202/270 11 70
www.beaschoenfeldt.de
info@beaschoenfeldt.de

Sandra Blumenthal
Alternative Health Practitioner
for Children and Adults
42369 Wuppertal-Ronsdorf
Phone: 0049 (0) 202/747 59 65
sandrab1975@hotmail.de

Uwe Haug
Alternative Health Practitioner
Unter Holzstr. 12
42653 Solingen
Phone: 0049 (0) 212/200 771
praxis@haug.it

Alternative Health Practitioner
Anita Burazin-Carapina
Marktstraße 8
46535 Dinslaken
Phone: 0049 (0) 2855/96 94 10
Mobile: 0049 (0) 173 591 80 26
www.carapina-anita.de
carapina@freenet.de

Monika Rekelhof
Alternative Animal Health Practitioner
Bedburger Str. 74
47574 Goch-Pfalzdorf
Phone: 0049 (0) 179 790 26 43
www.mobile-tierheilpraxis-monika.de
thp-klein@web.de

Christa Pohl
Health Advisor and Life Coach
Oesederstr. 103
49124 Georgsmarienhütte
Phone: 0049 (0) 171 211 73 87
christa.pohl@gmail.com

Postcode Area 5

Wilfried Kaufmann
Alternative Health Practitioner
Lindenstrasse 4
50674 Köln
Phone: 0049 (0) 221/240 21 57
www.naturheilpraxis-tao.de
info@naturheilpraxis-tao.de

Dr med. dent. Harald Werner
Dentist and Alternative Health Practitioner
Zülpicher Str. 2a
50674 Köln
Phone: 0049 (0) 221/923 12 94
www.za-dr-harald-werner.de
mail@za-dr-harald-werner.de

Irmgard Hilger
Alternative Health Practitioner
Finkenplatz 20
50735 Köln
Phone: 0049 (0) 221/712 59 59
Phone: 0049 (0) 221/712 44 96
Mobile: 0049 (0) 171 282 55 30
info@irmgard-hilger.de

Torsten Hagmaier
Alternative Health Practitioner
Praxis für Vitalität und Entgiftung
Kölner Strasse 80
51429 Bergisch Gladbach
Phone: 0049 (0) 2204/50 72 25
www.alternative-heilung.de
t.hagmaier@gmx.de

Dr rer. nat.
Alexandra Leffers-Knoll
Alternative Health Practitioner
Deutschherrenstr. 36
53177 Bonn
Phone: 0049 (0) 228/33 26 25
www.naturheilpraxis-leffers.de
lexilk@aol.com

Praxis für Naturheilverfahren
Yvonne Kallenberg und
Hans Joachim Freund
Heilpraktiker
Bahnhofsweg 3
56472 Fehl-Ritzhausen
Phone: 0049 (0) 2661/3803

Postcode Area 6

Steffi Rein
Energy Therapy for Animals
Ostertalstr. 14
66629 Freisen
Phone: 0049 (0) 177 37 38 870
www.energetik-sr.de
sr.mail69@web.de

Dr med. vet. Jan-Dirk Baumhäkel
Tierärztliche Praxis
Uhlandstr. 4
68647 Biblis
Phone: 0049 (0) 6245/7264

Rosemarie Heckmann
RSholistic ART
Auwiesen 4
69234 Dielheim
Phone: 0049 (0) 6222/318 02 98
Mobile: 0049 (0) 1520 170 38 17
www.rsholisticpraxis.jimdo.com
rosemarie.heckmann@email.de

Postcode Area 7

Martina Kistenfeger
Nurse
Walder Str. 14
72505 Krauchenwies
Phone: 0049 (0) 7576/92 99 570
m.kistenfeger@t-online.de

Appendix

Helmut Swoboda
Spiritual Healer
Billigheimer Str. 34
74861 Neudenau
Phone: 0049 (0) 6264/300
Fax: 06264/92 92 68
helmut.swoboda@t-online.de

Dr phil. Rosina Sonnenschmidt
Alternative Health Practitioner
Elisabethstr.1
75180 Pforzheim
rosinamaria@t-online.de
www.sonnenschmidt-knauss.de
rosinamaria@t-online.de

Katrin Gazdik
Alternative Health Practitioner
Jacob-Kast-Str. 24
76593 Gersbach
kgazdik@hotmail.de

Marcus Spitzfaden
Alternative Health Practitioner
Alte Bahnhofstrasse 21
76829 Landau
Phone: 0049 (0) 6341/994 96 70
Mobile: 0049 (0) 151 269 53 181
www.hp-spitzfaden.de
hp-spitzfaden@gmx.de

Raquel Reinert
Alternative Health Practitioner
Mühlweg 117
78054 Villingen-Schwenningen
Phone: 0049 (0) 7720/305 44 10
http://naturvita-erleben.de
info@naturvita-erleben.de

Marion Paar
Alternative Health Practitioner
Gewerbestr. 8a
79219 Staufen i. Br.
Phone: 0049 (0) 7633/945 90 39
www.naturheilpraxis-paar.de
mail@naturheilpraxis-paar.de

Stephanie Schöniger
Alternative Health Practitioner
Kastanienallee 28 f
76189 Karlsruhe
Phone: 0049 (0) 721/9767129
Fax: 0721/9767128
www.heilpraktikerin-hnc-karlsruhe.de
stephanie.schoeninger@gmail.com

Postcode Area 8

Manuela Schiffmann
HEILWEGE für Mensch & Tier
Alternative Health Practitioner and Healer
Weyarnerstr. 29
81547 München
Phone: 0049 (0) 89/699 79 468
www.heilwege.info

Karin Misar
Alternative Health Practitioner
Steinseestr. 3
81671 München
Phone: 0049 (0) 89/490 091 01
www.heilpraxis-karin-misar.de
post@heilpraxis-karin-misar.de

Beatrix Krause
Alternative Health Practitioner
Am Wasserbogen 2
82166 Gräfelfing
Phone: 0049 (0) 89/85 36 52
www.gesundheit-in-eigenverantwortung.de

Marlies Bader
Energy Healing for Humans and Animals
Breitackerweg 12
82491 Grainau
Phone: 0049 (0) 8821/1495
Marlies.Bader@gmx.de
www.energieheilarbeit-bader.de
www.tierheilpraxis-bader.de

Franz Wilhelm
Alternative Health Practitioner for Humans and Animals
Hochstr. 8
82544 Deining
Phone: 0049 (0) 8170/99 72 81
www.hochacht-direkt.de
franzwil@web.de

Veronika Wilczek
Alternative Health Practitioner
Finsterwalderstr. 3
83026 Rosenheim
Phone: 0049 (0) 8031/88 77 568
praxis-vw@go4more.de

Eva Geiger
Alternative Health Practitioner
Endorfer Str. 10
83083 Riedering
Phone: 0049 (0) 8036/908 51 64
geiger.globuli@gmx.de

Landpraxis für Naturheilverfahren
Alexandra Schwarz
Alternative Health Practitioner
Schröckerweg 9
83088 Kiefersfelden
Phone: 0049 (0) 8033/979 89 00

Andrea Schätz
Alternative Health Practitioner for Animals
Schulstraße 4
84533 Stammham
Phone: 0049 (0) 8678/749284

Praxis für ganzheitliche Medizin
Alternative Health Practitioner
Petra A. Kratschmann
Schloßangerweg 9
85635 Höhenkirchen
Phone: 0049 (0) 8102/729927
www.heilpraxis-kratschmann.de

Dr med. Walter A. Kratschmann
Facharzt für Allgemeinmedizin, Naturheilverfahren etc.
Schloßangerweg 9
85635 Höhenkirchen
Phone: 0049 (0) 8102/99 88 99
www.dr-kratschmann.de

Dr med. Beate Bruckner
Physiologische Tumortherapie
Biologischer Hormonausgleich
Hauptstr. 44
86405 Meitingen
Phone: 0049 (0) 8271/813 32 94
Fax: 08271/814 76 02
info@praxis-beate-bruckner.de

Albin Wirbel
Psychotherapist
Am Hang 21
87600 Kaufbeuren
Phone: 0049 (0) 8341/960 48 63
Mobile 0049 (0) 163 741 51 41
www.bewusst-sein-in-harmonie.de

Maria Zacherl
Alternative Health Practitioner
Dammweg 5
87616 Marktoberdorf
Phone: 0049 (0) 1577 386 6893
www.mariazacherl.de

Günther Hutter
Health Advisor
Von Behring Str. 6-8
88131 Lindau
guenther.hutter@gmail.com
Phone: 0049 (0) 043 650 55 55 856

Karin Rutka
Alternative Health Practitioner
Ingoldingerstr. 3
88427 Bad Schussenried
Phone: 0049 (0) 7583/2227
Mobile: 0049 (0) 171 185 04 04

Angela Surace
Alternative Health Practitioner
Nelly-Sachs-Str. 6
89134 Blaustein
Phone: 0049 (0) 731 950 1109
www.naturheilpraxis-surace.de
praxis@naturheilpraxis-surace.de

Postcode Area 9

Christian Hertel
Alternative Health Practitioner and Physiotherapist
Lederergasse 9
94032 Passau
Phone: 0049 (0) 851/966 66 58
hp-christian.hertel@gmx.net

Ingrid Probst
Alternative Health Practitioner
Friedmannsdorf 18
95239 Zell im Fichtelgebirge
Phone: 0049 (0) 9257/96 50 235
www.naturheilzentrum-probst.de
probst-ingrid@web.de

Sigrid Hotaki
Alternative Health Practitioner
Am Ölberg 5
96450 Coburg
Phone: 0049 (0) 049 (0) 9561/38080 (evenings)
waldzar@gmx.net

Appendix

Therapist for Psychosomatic Energetics
Alternative Health Practitioner
Carmen Fritz
An der Stadtmarter 32
97228 Rottendorf
Phone: 0049 (0) 9302/99 04 48
Mobile: 0049 (0) 170 432 25 89
carmen.fritz@t-online.de
www.pse-praxis-fritz.de

AUSTRIA

Maximilian Hoffmann
Präventologe
Stampfl 13
5570 Mauterndorf
Phone: 0043 (0) 664/530 94 09
max.hoffmann@sbg.at

Stefan Nagy
Energetiker
Kinderdorfstr. 15
9062 Moosburg
Phone: 0043 (0) 4272/83746
Mobile: 0043 (0) 676 700 51 91
s.nagy@aon.at

Harald Stempfl
Alternative Health Practitioner
Winterstellerweg 19
6380 St. Johann in Tirol
Phone: 0043 (0) 6991/508 55 90
www.mywa2balance.com
hst@myway2balance.com

Prof. Gerd Unterweger
Bio-Electric Healthcare Advisor
9584 Finkenstein
Schilfweg 2
Phone: 0043 (0) 676-680 63 68
lebewesentlich@draucom.at

SWITZERLAND

Heilpraxis
Martina-Annett Thaele-Franz
Heilpraktikerin
Hasen 39
6424 Lauerz (SZ)
Phone: 0041 (0) 511 2606
www.Heilpraktik-Thaele.ch
hp-thaele@sunrise.ch

Sabine Weber
Healthcare Advisor for Animals
Churfirstenblick 4
8758 Obstalden, GL
Phone: 0041 (0) 55/4121157
www.tiershiatsu-glarus.ch
weber.sabine@bluewin.ch

Ruth Frei
Alternative Health Practitioner
Hauptstrasse 79
9434 Au/St. Gallen
Phone: 0041 (0) 76/322 11 33
www.paranatura.li
bernstein@bluewin.ch

Index

Acid, excess 104, 120, 139, 146, 147
Acids and alkalines 19, 20, 21, 23, 28, 70, 103–104, 118, 170, 173, 174, 185, 208, 232
Acne 88, 122, 244
Actinic keratosis 88
Activator 36, 43, 54, 66, 83, 92–94, 95–99, 100, 101, 102, 103–104, 108, 111, 112, 115, 120, 121, 123, 124, 128–129, 131–132, 144–148, 151–152, 157, 158, 162, 164, 173, 186, 189, 191, 195–196
 – citric acid 32–33, 36, 55, 66, 82–83, 92, 94, 96–104, 115, 120, 123, 129, 133, 162, 164, 195–196
 – hydrochloric acid 23, 24, 92, 93, 94, 96, 97, 98, 99, 101, 102, 103, 104, 113, 115, 120, 123, 129, 145, 157, 162, 163, 195
 – instructions for activation 95–102
 – lemon juice, fresh 31, 97, 98, 99, 102, 103, 104, 131, 138
 – lime juice, fresh 97, 102
 – tartaric acid 92, 93, 94, 96, 97, 98, 101, 102, 103, 104, 115, 120, 123, 129, 141, 145, 148, 157, 162, 163, 195
Acupuncture 118, 188, 190, 217, 232
Age marks 34
Agglutination of red blood cells 155
AIDS 88, 153, 167, 176, 182
Akuamoa-Boateng, Dr Emmanuel 12, 264
Alexander Technique 170, 258
Alkalines and acids 19, 20, 21, 23, 28, 70, 103–104, 118, 170, 173, 174, 185, 208, 232
Allergic bronchopulmonary aspergillosis 88
Allergies 25, 36, 41, 52, 53, 76, 77, 88, 113, 114, 115, 116, 120, 157, 168, 204, 241, 242, 244, 252, 254, 270, 271, 274
Alpha hydroxy acid 240
Aluminium 168, 223, 240
Alzheimer's disease 88, 168, 223, 240
Amyotropic lateral sclerosis 88
Anaemia 88
Analgesia see Painkillers
Angina 88, 134
Animals, general 66, 81, 82, 83, 85, 86, 87, 137, 139, 143, 156, 160, 194–196, 228, 229, 230, 232, 240, 241, 243, 244
Animals, small 195
Ankylosing spondylitis (Bechterew's disease) 88
Anthrax (splenic fever) 88

Anticoagulants (Marcumar) 114, 120
Anti-inflammatories 75, 154, 155
Antioxidants 102, 197–200
Aphthous ulcer 58, 88
Apoplexy 88, 168, 189
Appendicitis 33
Apples 118, 120, 139
Arterial blockage 88
Arthritis 35, 88, 143, 169, 186
Art therapy 172
Asthma 35, 41, 53, 56, 88, 134, 171, 252
Athlete's foot 35, 41
Atopic dermatitis 52, 53, 122, 171, 215
Atrial fibrillation 88
Autism 65
Autogenic training 172, 188, 258
Awareness 171, 178, 207, 210, 258
Babies 109, 110, 122, 233, 234
Back problems 16, 49, 51, 88, 172, 218, 219
Bacterial prostatitis 88
Bad breath 74, 88, 126
Banis, Dr Ulrike 246
Bath additives, artificial 124
Bathing with MMS 80, 119, 123, 125, 175, 184, 188, 191
Bartonellosis 88
Batmanghelidj, Dr Fereydoon 224
Bee stings 44, 77
Belly aches see Stomach aches
Beta thalassaemia minor 88
Bioenergetics 170, 263
Biophotons 225–227, 231
Bipolar disorders 88
Birch, Kate 254
Bladder diseases 34, 61, 66–67, 88–89
Blood diseases 88
Blood pressure see Hypertension
Blood sedimentation, elevated 51
Blood-thinning medications 114, 120
Bone cancer 88
Bone, muscle and connective tissue pains 88
Bowel bacteria ESBL 34
Bowel diseases 89
Bowel parasites (giardia) 32
Breast cancer 88, 240, 242
Breast, inflammation of 89

Breath work 170, 258
Bronchitis 41, 49, 61, 88, 143
Bruising 38
Bruker, Dr Max Otto 232
Buchwald, Dr Gerhard 250, 254
Burns 25, 33, 88, 121, 173–174
Bursitis 88
Calves (animals) 86, 139, 196, 225
Cancer 25, 28, 33, 47, 51, 62, 67–70, 78, 88, 90–91, 122, 132, 150, 174–176, 185, 187–188, 197, 228, 233, 234, 240–243, 248
Candida infection 20, 46, 74, 92, 204
Cannula 111, 132, 145
Carpal Tunnel Syndrome 51, 88
Cataracts 88, 242
Cat hair allergy 88
CDS 12, 92, 100, 114, 137, 139, 140–144, 147–149, 160, 257
Chemical effect of MMS 23–29
Chemical reaction of MMS 23
Chickenpox 38, 88
Childhood diseases 177
Children 31, 36, 38, 40, 43, 44, 50, 65, 70, 95, 107–108, 111–112, 141, 152, 161, 162, 164–166, 177, 180, 217, 225, 233–234, 242, 244, 247, 248, 249, 252, 253
Chlorine allergy 113–114
Chlorine dioxide gas 24, 133–135, 138, 144–145, 162, 186
Chlorine dioxide solution 12, 92, 94, 112–113, 132, 133, 137–138, 139–144, 146, 147, 148, 149, 164, 204, 205
Chronic depression (dysthymia) 88
Chronic Fatigue Syndrome 88, 204
Chronic kidney diseases 88
Chronic lymphatic leukaemia 89
Chronic obesity 89
Chronic Pelvic Pain Syndrome (CPPS) 89
Circulation problems 35, 123, 155
Cirrhosis 89
Colds 40, 50, 51, 52, 59, 64, 74, 89, 109, 177
Collagen 240
Complaints after transplants 54, 88, 89, 154
Condyloma 89
Constipation 57, 65, 77
Contraindications 114–115, 132
Corns 143
Cosmetics 230, 238–239, 241, 243, 245
Coughs 38, 40, 41–42, 45, 49, 52, 64, 81
Coulter, Harris L. 254

Coxsackievirus 20, 177
Cramps 67, 89, 90
Craniosacral therapy 172
Crohn's disease 39, 89
Crystal orbs 248, 260
Cushing's disease 89
Cuts 38, 49, 183
Cystic fibrosis 89, 205
Cysts 35, 90, 205
Dandruff 67
Deacidification 118
Delarue, Simone 250–251
Dengue fever 89
Depression 43, 63, 88, 89, 219
Designer substances 232–233
Despopoulos, Agamemnon 221
Detoxification 26, 48, 51, 54, 67–68, 73, 78, 114, 119, 181, 191, 193, 240
Deutsches Ärzteblatt 178, 253
Diabetes Type 1 and 2 31, 49, 89, 177, 233, 234
Diarrhoea 13, 17, 47, 48, 49, 50, 51, 56, 67–68, 69, 71, 77, 83, 84, 86, 89, 100, 101, 108, 111, 112, 113, 116, 118, 128, 169, 180, 191, 194, 196, 205
Diethanolamine (DEA) 240
Diethyl phthalate 240
Digestive problems 41
Dioxychlor 132, 204–205
Discharge 35, 42, 67, 68, 82
Diuretics 154
Diverticulitis 89
DMSO 44–45, 80, 116, 154–159, 160, 161, 166, 168, 169, 188
Dog bites 58–59, 122
Doves 86, 196
Dry cough 52
Dysentery *see* Shigellosis
Earaches 89
Ear diseases 60, 73, 89, 196
Eczema 43, 67, 88, 89, 252
Edema *see* Oedemas
Effervescent tablets 137
Egoscue, Pete 170
Elastin with high relative molecular mass 240
Electrosmog 246, 248
Emotions / feelings 182, 210, 211, 213, 215, 217, 219, 236, 258
Emoto, Dr Masaru 224
Enema 126–128

Energetically imprinted globules 94, 100, 148–149, 172, 173, 183, 188, 260
Energy-saving bulbs 248–249
Erythema nodosum 89
European Parliament 253
Examples of use 96–102
Eye diseases and vision impairments 89, 129, 130, 179
Eye drops 12, 129–130, 179
Fahey, Trish 179, 234
Fasting 226
Feelings *see* Emotions
Feldenkrais 170, 187, 258
Ferreira, Peter 222, 224, 226
Fever 17, 38, 64, 71, 79, 88, 89, 110, 131, 186, 272
Fibromyalgia 40, 60, 89
Fischer, Dr Hartmut 12, 77, 112, 131, 132, 156, 159, 264
Fisher, Barbara L. 254
Flu (influenza) 20, 31, 40, 41, 50, 89, 109, 179, 180, 181, 186, 189, 192, 204, 252–254
Fluoride 241–242
Food 21, 39, 54, 67, 75, 93, 118, 138–139, 178–179, 198–199, 208, 210, 221, 223–234, 238
Food, disinfecting 138–139
Food, intolerances 52, 75, 80
Food, poisoning 89
Foot baths 38, 114, 116, 119, 128–129, 177, 181, 189
Formaldehyde /-donors 241, 244
Fungal infections 37, 40, 74, 80, 132, 204
Gas poisoning 114
Gas sack 136–137
Gastric ulcers 89
Gefeu solution 144–146, 148
Geopathic stress 246–248
Gittines, Roger 170
Glandular fever 71, 89
Gout 73, 74, 76, 89
Gray, John 236
Grimm, Hans-Ulrich 232–233
Haemorrhoids 35, 89
Hahnemann, Samuel 208
Hair problems 43, 54, 89
Hay fever 40, 89
Hay, Louise L. 172
Headaches 17, 73, 89, 91, 156, 186, 248, 249
Hearing, loss of 89, 190

Heart attack (DCM) 89
Heartburn 81, 89
Heart (cardiac) arrhythmias 88
Heart diseases 89, 181
Heart failure 54, 244
Heart palpitations 89, 177, 181
Heavy metals 13, 28, 37, 89, 108, 117, 192
Heavy metals, detox 192
Heavy metals, poisoning 89
Helicobacter infection 53, 89
Hendel, Dr Barbara 222, 224, 226
Hepatitis A, B, C and other hepatitis types 20, 25, 89, 181, 204
Herpes labialis and herpes zoster 89, 143, 182
Herxheimer reactions 131
Hesselink, Dr Thomas Lee 25, 29, 202
High blood pressure *see* Hypertension
HIV 25, 30, 89, 152, 182
Homeopathy 13, 67, 115, 118, 171, 184, 187, 208, 210, 218, 254, 260, 263–264
HPV (warts) 89
Hypertension (high blood pressure) 51, 54, 55, 182, 244
Hypochlorous acid 25, 28, 150–151, 153, 165
Immune system weakness 91, 205
Infants 38, 109–110, 215, 233, 250
Infections (all kinds) 13, 25, 34, 37, 39, 40, 41, 46, 47, 49, 50, 51, 53, 60, 61, 66, 67, 73, 74, 80, 82, 86, 89–92, 102, 109, 122, 128, 132, 134, 155, 186, 192, 194, 196, 204, 205, 208
Inflammations 35, 40–41, 43–44, 47, 50, 51, 58–59, 66, 74, 89, 122, 129, 134, 155, 177, 181, 215
Influenza *see* Flu
Infusions 39, 126, 130–133, 204–205
Injuries 25, 37, 57, 58, 74, 82, 154, 182–183, 249, 254
INR values 114
Insect bites 40, 122
Intestinal illnesses 32, 34, 39, 80, 89, 131
Iodine 59, 223
Irrigator 126–128
Irritable bladder 89
Irritable bowel 89
Itching 36, 38, 43, 46, 49, 53–54, 215–216
Jaw diseases 89
Joint pains 42, 76
Juices 31, 39, 40, 45, 63, 100–102, 106, 107, 109–112, 118, 140, 158, 167–168, 175, 177, 191, 197, 224, 230

Katie, Byron 211, 215
Kidney diseases 88, 89
Kidney failure 84, 89
Kidney infections 89
Kidney stones 89
Kidney under-function (renal insufficiency) 114
Kinesiology 52-53, 99, 171, 184, 188, 193, 209, 215-217
Knee pains 57
Koehof, Leo 11, 12, 55, 201, 206
Kremer, Dr Heinrich 176
Lacerations *see* Wounds
Lanolin 241
Large intestine diseases 89
Laryngitis 32
LD-50 values 160-161
Legs, nervous twitching, cramps in 90
Leishmaniasis 89
Leprosy 89
Leucocytosis 89
Leukaemia 89
Lichen sclerosis 53
Life rhythm 248
Light information 226
Light photons 226
Liver detox 116, 118, 119, 125, 176, 181, 191
Liver diseases 89, 114
Liver dysfunction 114
Lumbago 50
Lung infection 90, 205
Lung problems 90
Lupus erythematosus 90
Lyme disease 80, 90, 183-184
Lymphatic cancer 47
Lymphoma 90
Maes, Wolfgang 248-249
Maintenance dose 84, 102, 115, 168, 192-193
Malaria 17-19, 25-26, 30, 72, 78-79, 90, 91, 109, 110, 141, 184-185, 206
Marcumar 114, 120
Massage 55, 63, 124, 125, 170, 172
Meditation 69, 177, 256-257
Mega oesophagus 90
Melanoma 90, 185
Meningitis 90, 186
Metastasis 62, 88
Microorganisms 30, 31, 58, 108, 192
Microwaves 226

Middle ear infection 60, 73
Migraines 73, 90
Mindfulness *see* Awareness
Mineral oil 241
MMS
– discovery 19-22
– mixing 96
– overdose 68, 198
– protocols 11, 39, 50, 52, 77, 95-96, 100, 106-111, 113, 121, 122, 123, 125, 131, 143, 148, 152, 158, 167, 168, 169, 171, 172, 173, 174-176, 177, 179-180, 181, 182, 183, 185, 186, 187, 188, 189, 190, 193, 198, 202
– safety instructions for children, babies, pregnant women, animals, healthy people 160
– training courses 11, 202
MMS 1000 protocol 77-78, 106-107, 186
MMS 2 35, 116, 150-153, 160, 165, 168, 175, 180, 182, 184
MMS 2000 protocol 175, 187
Modified starch 233
Morgellons disease 90, 135, 137
Moritz, Andreas 71, 176,
Mosquito bites 79, 90
Mould infestations 92, 122, 135, 225, 232
Mouthwash 47, 61, 64
MRSA (Multiresistant Staphylococcus aureus) 54, 90, 185-187
Multiple myeloma (plasmacytoma) 90
Multiple sclerosis 90, 187
Muscle relaxation 155
Muscle tension 47, 90, 170
Music therapy 217
Myasthenia gravis 90
Mycoplasma diseases 20, 90, 204
Mycosis fungoides 90
Myomas 90
Nail diseases 90
Nanofilter 131, 132
Nausea threshold 123, 125, 128, 135, 175-176, 184, 191
Nervousness 90
Neuroendocrine tumours 91
Nilsson, Lennart 220
Nosebleeds 90
Nutrition 78, 93, 197-198, 225-226, 232-233
Oedemas 38, 90
Oesophagus diseases 90, 153
Operations 34, 44, 47, 50, 51, 52, 54, 62, 63, 70, 80, 114, 219-220

Organic seals 229
Osteopathy 170, 172, 217, 219
Osteopenia 90
Osteoporosis 90
Osteosarcoma 90
Ovarian cysts 90
Overacidification 80, 208–209
Overdose
 – sodium bicarbonate as antidote 119
 – vitamin C as antidote 119
Oversensitivity to various substances 90
Painkillers 43–45, 63
Pancreatic disorders 68–69, 90
Paralysis 43, 90–91
Parasites (also in pets) 19, 26, 32, 74, 75, 90, 136, 204
Parkinson's disease 90, 187
Parvovirus 20, 86, 90
Pearson, Leonard 179
Perfume 239, 241
Periodontitis 60, 64, 69
Photons 225–227, 231
pH-value 103–104, 131
Physiotherapy 44, 172, 217, 264
Pituitary tumours 90
Plants 66, 122, 231
Poisoning 26, 89, 90, 114, 186, 192
Pollen allergy 52, 76
Popp, Prof. Fritz-Albert 226–227, 231
Portal venous system 130
Pregnancies 38, 49, 89, 109
Preservatives 119, 137, 223, 227, 241
Preventative healthcare 49, 56, 70, 75, 82, 85, 193, 208, 250
Propylene glycol 242
Prostate conditions 33, 62, 77, 78, 90, 150
Psoriasis 33, 41, 90, 122
Psychotherapy 185, 209, 218–220, 260, 264, 265
Pulled muscles 183
Pyrogens 131
Q fever 90
Qi gong 170, 171, 188, 190, 258
Quick values 114, 120
Reactions 42, 99, 100, 108, 109, 110, 113, 114, 117, 118–120, 131, 143, 151, 156–157, 175, 180, 181, 183, 191, 193, 196
Recovery 36, 45, 71, 100, 165, 216
Relationship problems 236
Restless legs 90

Retinoblastomas 90
Rhinitis 36, 41, 143
Ringworm 122
Room cleansing 135
Rosacea 60
Rubella 90
Safety instructions 95, 111, 160–166
Salt 21–23, 54, 57, 72, 118, 124, 126–128, 160–161, 189, 221–224, 226
Sarcoidosis 90
Scarlet fever 90
Scarring 57, 90
Scheibner, Dr Viera 254
Sciatica 43, 90
Scoliosis 90
Seasickness 60
Serious illnesses 91, 109, 131, 143, 182, 198
Severely ill patients 131
Sexually transmitted diseases 90
Shigellosis 90
Shingles (herpes zoster) 89, 182
Side effects 22, 32, 34, 36, 37, 39, 44, 47, 48, 66, 118, 132, 156, 185, 205, 251, 253
Silbernagl, Stefan 221
Simonton, O. Carl 176, 177, 220
Singing 170, 172
Sinus, fungal infection in 89
Sinusitis 13, 41, 89, 90, 143
Skin cancer 122, 185, 188
Skin diseases 53, 90, 122, 171, 188
Skin eruptions (rash) 38, 215, 241
Skin impurities 74, 90
Slow activation based on the Fischer method 12, 77–78, 112–113, 146, 148, 181, 189
Snoring 51
Soap 123–124, 128, 162, 164, 165, 239, 245
Sodium bicarbonate 12, 72, 104–106, 112–113, 117, 119–120, 147, 162
Sodium fluoride 242
Sodium laureth sulphate 242
Sodium lauryl sulphate 242
Softening agents 121, 233–234
SOMA therapy 170, 172, 217
Spinal stenosis 90
Spots 37, 42, 43, 45, 47, 72–73, 90
Sprains 183
Stoichiometric calculation 132
Stokes, Gordon 217
Stomach aches 45, 48, 68, 152
Stomach cramps 90

Stroke *see* Apoplexy
Studies 24, 26, 156, 178–179, 206, 219, 226, 228, 240, 242, 247, 250, 252–254
Sunburn 174, 189
Sunscreen filter 242
Swine flu *see* Flu
Syringe, single-use 37, 87, 111, 128, 131–132, 145, 194–195
Tai chi 189
Talc 243
Tapeworm infections 90
Taste enhancers 230
Teeth 33, 38–39, 55, 60, 63, 64, 66, 74, 125–126, 134–135, 225
Temelie, Barbara 234
Tension headaches 91
Tetanus 91, 250–252
Thinking, concentration and memory disorders 91
Thoughts 69, 171–172, 210–220, 235, 256
Thrombocyte aggregation inhibitors 155
Thrombocytopenia 91
Thyroid disorders 46–47, 77, 91
Time management 237
Tinnitus 91, 189–190
Tiredness 91, 221
Toiletries and cosmetics 230, 238–239, 241, 243, 245
Toxins 28, 73, 74, 116, 119, 125, 192, 241
Toxoplasmosis 46
Traditional Chinese Medicine (TCM) 189
Transplants, subsequent complaints 54, 88, 89, 154
Trigeminal neuralgia 63, 91
Tuberculosis (TB) 20, 32, 56, 90, 204, 250
Tumours, cancerous and non-cancerous 26, 44, 50, 51, 57, 81, 83, 90, 91, 176, 239
Turnaround 211–214
Typhus 15, 17, 91
Ulcerative colitis 91
Ureter diseases 91
Varicose veins 54, 65, 91
Vegetable capsules 111, 150
Vegetarianism 228, 232
Venous ulcers (on legs) 91
Viruses 20, 21, 25, 37, 39, 46, 71, 86, 89, 90, 132, 155, 177, 181, 204, 209, 253
Vitamin C, general 107, 115, 175, 197–200
 – as an antidote to MMS 119
 – avoid overdoses in juices 100–102
 – beneficial for arterial walls 169

Vitamin E 198–199
Vocal cord paralysis 91
Vomiting 70, 71, 84, 116, 120, 162, 163, 164, 180, 186
Warts 34, 40, 46, 56, 89, 91, 122, 143
Water, drinking 15, 22, 24, 51, 68, 81, 86, 92, 93, 151, 204–205, 223
 – preparation 22, 24, 137–138
 – quality 22
 – requirements 223–224
Weakness, physical 44, 71, 91, 205
Weather, sensitivity to (Meteoropathy) 64, 90, 177
Wegener's granulomatosis 89
Weight, excess 50, 52, 59, 83, 89, 178–179, 233–234
Whiteside, Daniel 217
Whooping cough 38, 252
Wolcott, William L. 179, 234
Wounds 40, 43, 49, 52, 55, 58, 59, 62, 74, 80, 122, 124, 155, 173, 182, 215
Yeast infections 91
Yellow fever 91
Yoga 170, 171, 189, 258
Zilgrei 170, 172, 258
Zurhorst, Eva-Maria 236

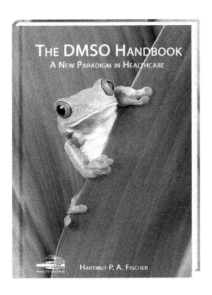

The DMSO Handbook

by

Dr. rer. nat. Hartmut Fischer

DMSO, an easily accessible universal therapeutic agent, is currently enjoying a remarkable comeback in the field of alternative medicine after having been treasured for many years by just a small number of insiders. It has mainly become known as a fast-acting, well-tolerated treatment for acute inflammations and traumatic injuries. It has an anti-inflammatory effect, it relieves pain immediately, it accelerates the swift resorption of swellings and haemorrhages, and it supports wound healing. But DMSO does much more. This natural substance is an extremely useful basis for therapeutic self-reliance and a huge leap towards freedom from the many side effects caused by standard medications.

Dr Hartmut Fischer is a scientist and alternative health practitioner. In this book, he draws upon many years of experience of working with DMSO, both in a scientific capacity as well as in his role as a health professional.

292 pages. Hardback. ISBN 978-3-9815255-1-9

For more information visit www.daniel-peter-verlag.de

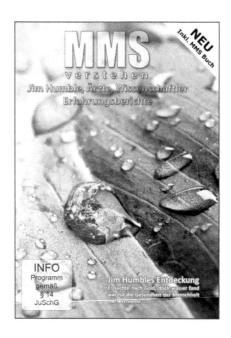

The documentary film
MMS verstehen / Understanding MMS
on DVD
fourth revised edition!

Audio in English / German / Spanish

This film imparts a deeper understanding of MMS. It features doctors, scientists and users, and you will meet in it some of the people mentioned in The MMS Handbook, such as Jim Humble, Dr John Humiston and Clara Beltrones.

The efficacy of MMS is documented using numerous first-hand reports. It is truly inspiring to learn how people have used MMS to cure serious and refractory illnesses.

Now in a fourth revised edition with:

– a 16-page booklet (in German only) which includes interesting articles on MMS, and detailed usage instructions for the most common MMS sets on the market today

– a bonus video on structured water and the surprising effect of structured water on plants.

Format DVD9. Playing time: 105 minutes. Languages: English, German, Spanish.   ISBN 978-3-9812917-0-4

For more information visit www.daniel-peter-verlag.de

www.ingramcontent.com/pod-product-compliance
Lightning Source LLC
LaVergne TN
LVHW082122110125
801043LV00005B/43